# The Vision of the Future of Obstetrics & Gynecology

*Editors*

DENISSE S. HOLCOMB
F. GARY CUNNINGHAM

## OBSTETRICS AND GYNECOLOGY CLINICS OF NORTH AMERICA

www.obgyn.theclinics.com

*Consulting Editor*
WILLIAM F. RAYBURN

December 2021 • Volume 48 • Number 4

**ELSEVIER**

1600 John F. Kennedy Boulevard • Suite 1800 • Philadelphia, Pennsylvania, 19103-2899

http://www.theclinics.com

OBSTETRICS AND GYNECOLOGY CLINICS OF NORTH AMERICA Volume 48, Number 4
December 2021 ISSN 0889-8545, ISBN-13: 978-0-323-81353-2

Editor: Kerry Holland
Developmental Editor: Hannah Almira Lopez

*Obstetrics and Gynecology Clinics* (ISSN 0889-8545) is published quarterly by Elsevier Inc., 360 Park Avenue South, New York, NY 10010-1710. Months of issue are March, June, September, and December. Periodicals postage paid at New York, NY, and additional mailing offices. Subscription price per year is $335.00 (US individuals), $944.00 (US institutions), $100.00 (US students), $404.00 (Canadian individuals), $991.00 (Canadian institutions), $100.00 (Canadian students), $459.00 (international individuals), $991.00 (international institutions), and $225.00 (international students). To receive student/resident rate, orders must be accompanied by name of affiliated institution, date of term, and the signature of program/residency coordinator on institution letterhead. Orders will be billed at individual rate until proof of status is received. Foreign air speed delivery is included in all *Clinics* subscription prices. All prices are subject to change without notice. POSTMASTER: Send address changes to *Obstetrics and Gynecology Clinics*, Elsevier Health Sciences Division, Subscription Customer Service, 3251 Riverport Lane, Maryland Heights, MO 63043. **Customer Service: Telephone: 1-800-654-2452 (U.S. and Canada); 314-447-8871 (outside U.S. and Canada). Fax: 314-447-8029. E-mail: journalscustomerservice-usa@elsevier.com (for print support); journalsonlinesupport-usa@elsevier. com (for online support).**

*Reprints.* For copies of 100 or more of articles in this publication, please contact the Commercial Reprints Department, Elsevier Inc., 360 Park Avenue South, New York, New York 10010-1710. Tel.: 212-633-3874; Fax: 212-633-3820; E-mail: reprints@elsevier.com.

*Obstetrics and Gynecology Clinics of North America* is also published in Spanish by McGraw-Hill Interamericana Editores S.A., P.O. Box 5-237, 06500, Mexico; in Portuguese by Reichmann and Affonso Editores, Rio de Janeiro, Brazil; and in Greek by Paschalidis Medical Publications, Athens, Greece.

*Obstetrics and Gynecology Clinics of North America is* covered in *MEDLINE/PubMed (Index Medicus), Excerpta Medica, Current Concepts/Clinical Medicine, Science Citation Index, BIOSIS, CINAHL, and ISI/BIOMED.*

# Contributors

## CONSULTING EDITOR

**WILLIAM F. RAYBURN, MD, MBA**
Adjunct Professor, Department of Obstetrics and Gynecology, College of Graduate Studies, Medical University of South Carolina, Charleston, South Carolina; Associate Dean, Continuing Medical Education and Professional Development, Distinguished Professor and Emeritus Chair, Professor, Maternal Fetal Medicine, Department of Obstetrics and Gynecology, University of New Mexico School of Medicine, Albuquerque, New Mexico

## EDITORS

**DENISSE S. HOLCOMB, MD**
Assistant Professor, Department of Obstetrics and Gynecology, The University of Texas Southwestern Medical Center, Dallas, Texas

**F. GARY CUNNINGHAM, MD**
Department of Obstetrics and Gynecology, The University of Texas Southwestern Medical Center, Dallas, Texas

## AUTHORS

**ARNOLD P. ADVINCULA, MD**
Professor and Chief, Gynecologic Specialty Surgery, Columbia University Irving Medical Center, New York, New York

**ERIC BERGH, MD**
Assistant Professor, Department of Obstetrics and Gynecology, The Fetal Center at Children's Memorial Hermann Hospital, The University of Texas Health Science Center at Houston, McGovern Medical School, Houston, Texas

**CARA BUSKMILLER, MD**
Fellow, Maternal Fetal Medicine, Department of Obstetrics and Gynecology, The University of Texas Health Science Center at Houston, McGovern Medical School, Houston, Texas

**FRANK A. CHERVENAK, MD**
Professor and Chair, Department of Obstetrics and Gynecology, Donald and Barbara Zucker School of Medicine at Hofstra/Northwell and Lenox Hill Hospital, New York, New York

**SHENA DILLON, MD**
Assistant Professor, Department of Obstetrics and Gynecology, The University of Texas Southwestern Medical Center, Dallas, Texas

**KEVIN J. DOODY, MD**
Director, CARE Fertility, Bedford, Texas; Clinical Professor, The University of Texas Southwestern Medical Center, Dallas, Texas

**ALLISON L. GILBERT, MD, MPH**
Co-Medical Director, Southwestern Women's Surgical Center, Dallas, Texas

**MEADOW MAZE GOOD, DO, FACOG**
Physician Advisor, ABOG Board Certified in Obstetrics and Gynecology and Female Pelvic Medicine and Reconstructive Surgery, Winnie Palmer Hospital for Women and Babies, OrlandoHealth, Orlando, Florida

**ESTHER S. HAN, MD, MPH**
Fellow, Minimally Invasive Gynecologic Surgery, Columbia University Irving Medical Center, New York, New York

**BARBARA L. HOFFMAN, MD**
Distinguished Professor in Obstetrics and Gynecology, in Honor of F. Gary Cunningham, M.D., Professor, Department of Obstetrics and Gynecology, The University of Texas Southwestern Medical Center, Dallas, Texas

**DENISSE S. HOLCOMB, MD**
Assistant Professor, Department of Obstetrics and Gynecology, The University of Texas Southwestern Medical Center, Dallas, Texas

**ANTHONY JOHNSON, MD**
Professor, Department of Obstetrics and Gynecology, The Fetal Center at Children's Memorial Hermann Hospital, The University of Texas Health Science Center at Houston, McGovern Medical School, Houston, Texas

**JESSICA LEE, MD, FACOG**
Assistant Professor, Division of Gynecologic Oncology, Department of Obstetrics and Gynecology, The University of Texas Southwestern Medical Center, Dallas, Texas

**LAURENCE B. McCULLOUGH, PhD**
Professor, Department of Obstetrics and Gynecology, Donald and Barbara Zucker School of Medicine at Hofstra/Northwell and Lenox Hill Hospital, New York, New York

**NAVYA NAIR, MD, MPH, FACOG**
Assistant Professor, Division of Gynecologic Oncology, Department of Obstetrics and Gynecology, LSU Health Sciences Center – New Orleans, New Orleans, Louisiana

**WILLIAM F. RAYBURN, MD, MBA**
Adjunct Professor, Department of Obstetrics and Gynecology, College of Graduate Studies, Medical University of South Carolina, Charleston, South Carolina; Associate Dean, Continuing Medical Education and Professional Development, Distinguished Professor and Emeritus Chair, Professor, Maternal Fetal Medicine, Department of Obstetrics and Gynecology, University of New Mexico School of Medicine, Albuquerque, New Mexico

**STACI TANOUYE, MD, FACOG**
Physician, ABOG Board Certified in Obstetrics and Gynecology, Women's Care of Florida, Jacksonville, Florida

**IMAM M. XIERALI, PhD**
Associate Professor, Department of Family and Community Medicine, The University of Texas Southwestern Medical Center, Dallas, Texas

# Contents

> Simulation in obstetrics and gynecology has advanced significantly since its beginnings in the seventeenth century with wooden birthing and pelvic models. In recent years, more and more evidence has emerged showing improvements in participant confidence, skills, behaviors, and, finally, patient outcomes following simulation program implementation. Several regulatory bodies and national organizations have begun to require simulation of obstetrician-gynecologists, and the newer generation of physicians has experienced simulation throughout their training. Simulation is embedded in the medical culture and hopefully is making obstetrician-gynecologists better for it.

> Gynecologic cancers contribute to a significant portion of cancer morbidity and mortality among women in the United States and across the globe. This article provides a comprehensive review of current screening guidelines and novel techniques that have promise in the prevention and early detection of gynecologic cancers in the future. The authors anticipate a move toward less invasive testing modalities, use of cancer biomarkers, and the prevention and treatment of high-risk factors such as human papilloma virus infection and obesity.

> Many sexually active, reproductive-aged persons capable of becoming pregnant use some method of contraception. To expand options for those desiring birth control, new choices include a vaginal ring, transdermal patch, progestin-only pill, and spermicide. Compared with currently available methods, additional technologies that are highly effective, easy to use, cost efficient, and well-tolerated lay on the horizon. During contraceptive counseling, patient choice, and reproductive autonomy should remain paramount.

The growth in the number of obstetrics and gynecology resident graduates pursuing fellowships has exceeded growth in the number of resident graduates, because more fellowship programs are being developed in more subspecialties rather than additional residency programs. Approximately 1 in 4 residents pursues subspecialty training, compared with 1 in 12 in 2001. The number of fellowships remains competitive, because nearly all programs fill their match and the number of applicants exceeds the number of positions. Graduating residents who serve as frontline women's health specialists need to serve as leaders of interprofessional teams to better serve their patients, especially in underserved areas.

The field of fetal medicine has evolved significantly over the past several decades. Our ability to identify and treat the unborn patient has been shaped by advancements in imaging technology, genetic diagnosis, an improved understanding of fetal physiology, and the development and optimization of in utero surgical techniques. The future of the field will be shaped by medical innovators pushing for the continued refinement of minimally invasive surgical technique, the application of pioneering technologies such as robotic surgery and in utero stem cell and gene therapies, and the development of innovative ex utero fetal support systems.

Robotics has become an essential part of the surgical armamentarium for a growing number of surgeons around the world. New companies seek to compete with established robotic systems that have dominated the market to date. Evolving robotic surgery platforms have introduced technologic and design advancements to optimize ergonomics, improve visualization, provide haptic feedback, and make systems smaller and cheaper. With the introduction of any new technology in the operating room, it is imperative that safeguards be in place to ensure its appropriate use. Current processes for granting of hospital robotic surgery privileges are inadequate and must be strengthened and standardized.

Fetal analysis uses noninvasive and invasive methods to obtain images and tissues for interpretation that supports risk assessment and/or diagnosis of the fetus's condition. This article provides ethically justified, clinically applicable guidance for supporting the pregnant patient's decision making about fetal analysis. Topics include ethical reasoning using key ethical concepts, confidentiality, clarity about the pregnant woman as ultimate decision maker, offering fetal analysis, counseling about results, counseling about accepted maternal-fetal intervention, and counseling about innovation and research on maternal-fetal intervention. Professional ethics is an essential component of counseling pregnant patients about fetal analysis and referral for investigative maternal-fetal intervention.

## Social Media Superpowers in Obstetrics and Gynecology    787

Meadow Maze Good and Staci Tanouye

This article encourages the obstetrician-gynecologists to use social media platforms to share their wealth of clinical expertise and experience with the public in an engaging and empowering way. Social media is a powerful tool that increases communication, education, and support that can be leveraged to increase comprehension of women's health topics and advocate for our patients, both inside and outside the examination room. Included are tips for physicians on how to harness their social media superpower to connect with patients on social media, build a brand, and network in a meaningful and authentic way.

## Infertility Treatment Now and in the Future    801

Kevin J. Doody

Treatment of infertility has evolved as understanding of reproduction has improved. Fertility promoting surgery still is performed and recent advances have broken new ground. Hormonal treatments to correct gonadal dysfunction have been developed, but multiple gestation continues to be a significant complication. Assisted reproductive technologies have improved such that in vitro fertilization and its variants increasingly are used to treat nearly all causes of infertility. Advances in assisted reproduction are of 2 types: (1) incremental optimization of existing techniques and (2) development of new, disruptive technologies. Artificial intelligence and stem cell technologies are poised to have impact in the near future.

## Postscript: Women's Health and the Era After COVID-19    813

Denisse S. Holcomb and William F. Rayburn

As the world clamored to respond to the rapidly evolving coronavirus 2019 (COVID-19) pandemic, health care systems reacted swiftly to provide uninterrupted care for patients. Within obstetrics and gynecology, nearly every facet of care was influenced. Rescheduling of office visits, safety of labor and delivery and in the operating room, and implementation of telemedicine are examples. Social distancing has impacted academic centers in the education of trainees. COVID-19 vaccine trials have increased awareness of including pregnant and lactating women. Last, the pandemic has reminded us of issues related to ethics, diversity and inclusiveness, marginalized communities, and the women's health workforce.

# OBSTETRICS AND GYNECOLOGY CLINICS

**SERIES OF RELATED INTEREST**

*Clinics in Perinatology*
www.perinatology.theclinics.com
*Pediatric Clinics of North America*
https://www.pediatrics.theclinics.com

**THE CLINICS ARE AVAILABLE ONLINE!**
Access your subscription at:
www.theclinics.com

# Foreword

# Learning from the Past for a Better Future in Women's Health Care

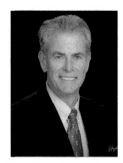

William F. Rayburn, MD, MBA
*Consulting Editor*

This issue of the *Obstetrics and Gynecology Clinics of North America* is a vision into the future of several issues affecting obstetricians-gynecologists. Edited by Denisse Sanchez Holcomb, MD and Gary Cunningham, MD from the University of Texas Southwestern Medical Center in Dallas, Texas, the readers become aware of the expansion in knowledge from the distant and recent past. Advancements in contraceptive technology, infertility, fetal diagnostic testing and surgery, early screening of gynecologic cancers, and robotic surgery are examples highlighted in this issue. Education is also featured in articles pertaining to simulation and the future of social media in our daily practices. Physician practices are reviewed by examining subspecialization in our field and how it affects access to women's health care in the future.

As I reviewed these articles, I reflected on the spirit, resilience, and creativity of the women's health community during these past few years. Facing unprecedented challenges from the COVID-19 pandemic, providers adapted rapidly and efficiently, offering critical collaboration with others to respond to the public health crisis. Many demonstrated strength and compassion despite economic losses and reductions in the number of clinic options. Undoubtedly, this increased engagement with other health care professionals will serve us well into the future.

It was a pleasure for me to coauthor a postscript with Dr Holcomb about the effect of COVID-19 on our future delivery of women's health care and the need to care for ourselves. Many of you suffered personal illness and grieved the loss of loved ones and colleagues, while contending with stress and change in your work environment. As we reflect on this experience, you should note your ability to rise to the challenges we will continue to face. We leveraged teamwork to endure these difficult experiences, and we will meet the upcoming challenges together with the same spirit in the future.

Obstet Gynecol Clin N Am 48 (2021) xi–xii
https://doi.org/10.1016/j.ogc.2021.07.006
0889-8545/21/© 2021 Published by Elsevier Inc.

obgyn.theclinics.com

As we envision the future, adjustments to changing times will be essential for women's health care teams. I look forward to learning more about effectively addressing ongoing challenges, including medical misinformation, distrust of science, physician burnout, and health equity and disparities. Dr Holcomb, Dr Cunningham, and their team of experienced authors brought timely, thoughtful, and occasionally provocative insights about the topics mentioned above. Regardless of whether a woman's health care is provided by an obstetrician-gynecologist alone or in conjunction with other qualified providers, it is important to clearly demonstrate the power of education and performance to make our patients healthier while living in a better place.

William F. Rayburn, MD, MBA
Department of Obstetrics and Gynecology
University of New Mexico School of Medicine
MSC 10 5580, 1 University of New Mexico
Albuquerque, NM 87131-0001, USA

*E-mail address:*
wrayburnmd@gmail.com

# Preface
# Seeing Past the Horizon

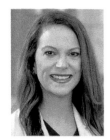 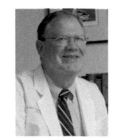

Denisse S. Holcomb, MD    F. Gary Cunningham, MD
*Editors*

We would like to welcome you to this issue of *Obstetrics and Gynecology Clinics of North America* entitled, "A Vision of the Future of Obstetrics and Gynecology."

In our daily lives as obstetrician-gynecologists, we may sometimes take for granted the discoveries of predecessors that paved the path for the way we practice today. Every moment spent scrubbing before surgeries, we do not stop to consider the groundbreaking work by Ignaz Semmelweis that allowed this act to become so commonplace today.[1] When we turn to obstetrical forceps during prolonged second-stage labors, it is unlikely that our thoughts should wander to the ingenuity of the Chamberlen brothers.[2] Yet, if it were not for impactful technological advancements such as these, our field would not be where it is today.

The purpose of this issue is twofold: (1) To consider how we have arrived at our current standards within various aspects of obstetrics and gynecology, and (2) to speculate where the future will take us.

In this issue, we have asked authors to report how different aspects of our field will continue to evolve in the future. Topics include the future of gynecologic cancer screening, emerging contraceptive technologies, robotic surgery, fetal surgery, treating infertility, and simulation in obstetrics and gynecology. We explore the ever-evolving use of social media in medicine, the ethics of prenatal genetic diagnosis techniques, future trends in subspecialization within our field, and even life after COVID-19.

Obstet Gynecol Clin N Am 48 (2021) xiii–xiv
https://doi.org/10.1016/j.ogc.2021.07.002
0889-8545/21/© 2021 Published by Elsevier Inc.

obgyn.theclinics.com

We hope that these articles will be thought-provoking and provide special insights into emerging technologies within our field.

Denisse S. Holcomb, MD
University of Texas Southwestern
Medical Center in Dallas
Department of Obstetrics and Gynecology
5939 Harry Hines Boulevard
Dallas, TX 75390, USA

F. Gary Cunningham, MD
University of Texas Southwestern
Medical Center in Dallas
Department of Obstetrics and Gynecology
5323 Harry Hines Boulevard
Dallas, TX 75390-9032, USA

*E-mail addresses:*
denisse.holcomb@utsouthwestern.edu (D.S. Holcomb)
gary.cunningham@utsouthwestern.edu (F.G. Cunningham)

## REFERENCES

1. Kadar N. Rediscovering Ignaz Philipp Semmelweis (1818-1865). Am J Obstet Gynecol 2019;220(1):26–39.
2. Baskett TF. Operative vaginal delivery—an historical perspective. Best Pract Res Clin Obstet Gynaecol 2019;56:3–10.

# Simulation in Obstetrics and Gynecology

## A Review of the Past, Present, and Future

Shena Dillon, MD

### KEYWORDS

- Simulation • Patient safety • Obstetrics • Gynecology • Team training

### KEY POINTS

- Simulation has a long history in obstetrics and gynecology and now is ubiquitous in training programs across the country.
- Research supports using simulation for skills training and to improve teamwork and communication.
- As such, it has become a mainstay of safe patient care in obstetrics and gynecology.

## INTRODUCTION

Simulation has become a mainstay of safe culture in medicine since *To Err is Human* brought to light how far the medical community needed to go to improve patient safety.[1] By providing a safe environment for medical practitioners to learn from mistakes, simulation has been shown to advance medical knowledge and team dynamics, both of which are equally important for preventing errors in patient care.[2–5] Simulation itself has developed into its own specialty of medicine, with fellowships in simulation widely available in many specialties.[6] The field of obstetrics and gynecology has a long history of incorporating simulation into teaching of medical knowledge and surgical skills but is relatively young compared with other specialties in its adoption of team-based exercises for obstetric and gynecologic emergencies as well as incorporation of newer technology into surgical training.[7,8] The purpose of this review is to highlight how far simulation has come in both the obstetric and gynecologic fields and predict where it is headed in the future.

## DEFINITIONS IN SIMULATION

Before embarking on a discussion regarding simulation, it is important to distinguish terms related to the field because simulation takes on many different meanings

The author has nothing to disclose.
Department of Obstetrics and Gynecology, University of Texas Southwestern Medical Center, 5323 Harry Hines Boulevard, Dallas, TX 75390-9032, USA
*E-mail address:* shena.dillon@utsouthwestern.edu

Obstet Gynecol Clin N Am 48 (2021) 689–703
https://doi.org/10.1016/j.ogc.2021.07.003
0889-8545/21/© 2021 Elsevier Inc. All rights reserved.
obgyn.theclinics.com

depending on the desired outcome of the experience. First and foremost, a simulator is any physical object, device, situation, or environment where a task or series of tasks can be represented realistically.[9] This definition can encompass something as basic as a bony pelvis with a cloth baby or as complex as a simulation center with spaces made to mimic real-life operating rooms. Simulators that serve as the patient often are referred to as manikins.[10] Next, when discussing simulation activities, it is important to distinguish between procedural simulation, or task trainers, and full-immersion clinical simulation.[11] Procedural simulation typically refers to tasks performed by a single individual in a short amount of time with the main function of assessing adequacy of a particular skill. This can be done in a variety of clinical or educational environments with relatively inexpensive simulators allowing for real-time skill assessment prior to performing the actual procedure. An example is a shoulder dystocia drill using a pelvis model and cloth baby to practice maneuvers to relieve the dystocia while awaiting delivery of an infant with suspected macrosomia. In contrast, full-immersion clinical simulation involves performance of a complex set of tasks in a realistic health care setting with several team members interacting with each other and a standardized patient or manikin. This type of simulation typically is conducted by a team of simulationists who have prepared for weeks, or sometimes months or years, in advance in order to replicate the clinical environment as closely as possible to real life. When discussing how closely simulation mimics real life, fidelity, or the realness of the simulator, is an important component (**Table 1**). Low-fidelity simulators are less like the real-life situation and typically are less expensive. In contrast, high-fidelity simulators are more expensive and use more advanced technology to try to replicate real life. A third type of simulator is the hybrid model, which involves a human actor (sometimes referred to as a confederate) wearing a simulator while performing the part of the patient. Although it may seem intuitive that high-fidelity simulation is superior, the literature has shown benefits from all 3 types of simulation.[12,13] Finally, a newer branch of simulation uses virtual reality (VR) as the simulator.[14] This immersive experience mimics game-based learning that is familiar to today's younger generation of obstetrician/gynecologists and is more like full-immersion simulation in experience but can be done by a single individual on their own time like a procedural trainer.

The activities surrounding the simulation event are just as important, some would say even more important, as the simulation itself; they have their own definitions as

**Table 1**
**Types of simulators**

|  | Personnel Involved | Environment | Fidelity | Expense |
|---|---|---|---|---|
| Task trainer | Participant only; may require an observer | Any location | Low to medium | $–$$ |
| Full-body manikin | Usually several participants to form a team and simulationists | Full-immersion clinical simulation typically in a simulation center | High | $$$ |
| Hybrid | Patient-actor and participant; team may be involved | Full-immersion clinical simulation | Medium | $–$$ |
| VR | Participant only | Full-immersion clinical simulation created by device (center not necessary) | High | $$$ |

well. The prebrief is the time spent before the simulation begins when the person or team conducting the simulation explain the rules of the simulation environment and what is expected of the team, including gaps in fidelity and how long the simulation should last before ending.[15] This also is the time to describe and espouse the basic assumption, which is the belief held by the simulation team conducting the experience that all participants are smart and capable health care team members who desire to do what is best for their patients and strive to improve their care toward this goal.[16] This step is crucial in any simulation activity but especially critical in team environments, to protect the psychological safety of simulation participants. Only when participants feel safe can they learn from mistakes without fear of judgment. Following the prebrief is the simulation itself, which then is followed by the debrief.[17–19] The debriefing time is where most simulationists feel the power of simulation lies. This is when participants reflect on what happened during the experience and analyze how certain aspects can be improved. This reflection and analysis allow for retention of knowledge in adult learners in ways that traditional didactic learning cannot, which then can lead to improved patient care as well as identification of system issues not commonly shared during real-life scenarios. Skilled debriefing allows participants to drive the discussion with open communication and leaning toward curiosity and away from judgment.[18] Establishing the basic assumption in the prebrief is paramount for success in the debrief. Following a successful debrief, the hope is that simulation participants go back into their clinical environments with skills learned and retained from the simulation.

## HISTORIC CONTEXT

Having established basic definitions for language pertaining to simulation, its history in both obstetrics and gynecology can be reviewed. The first simulators recorded in obstetrics dates back to the ninth century, where small wooden figures were used to demonstrate childbirth.[20] This was followed by dearth of new developments until the seventeenth century, when newer simulators called phantoms were used to teach midwives how to manage difficult birthing scenarios.[21] Shortly thereafter, Gregoire the Elder and his son fashioned a newer phantom out of wicker and used a dead child to teach similar maneuvers. This led to the development of a pelvis simulator model created from human bones covered by leather accompanied by a fetus made of wood and rubber by Sir William Smellie, father of British midwifery, innovator of forceps design and part of the trio who invented the Mauriceau-Smellie-Veit maneuver for breech delivery.[22] Others made further advancements in phantoms of that time, including a glass version by Sir Richard Manningham and a wicker-fabric-leather-sponge version by Madame du Coudray, called "the Machine," which is on display in the Louvre today (**Fig. 1**).[20,23] In the nineteenth century, Professor B.S. Schulze created a pelvic floor model with interchangeable cervical dilations and bony structures to aid practitioners in determining adequacy of the pelvis.[24] The next obstetric simulator of note was developed by Knapp and Eades[25] in the 1970s and featured mechanical parts that simulated vaginal birth (**Fig. 2**). This represented a leap forward in the obstetric simulation world in terms of technological advancement and shortly followed the development of the SimOne manikin by anesthesiologists at the University of Southern California in the 1960s.[26] although the vaginal birth simulator by Knapp and Eades was controlled by cranks and levers, SimOne, created by Drs Denson and Abrahamson, was the first computer-controlled patient simulator that allowed for intubation and central line placement as well as other realistic aspects of a code blue scenario. Twenty years later, Eggert, Eggert, and Vallejo created an obstetric version of a full patient manikin with a motorized mechanism for pushing called Noelle (Gaumard

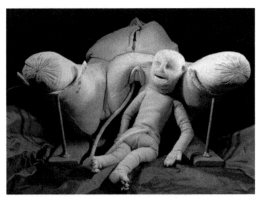

**Fig. 1.** The Machine obstetric simulator of Madame du Coudray. (*Courtesy of* Musée Flaubert et d'histoire et de la médecine – CHU de Rouen, Rouen, France; with permission.)

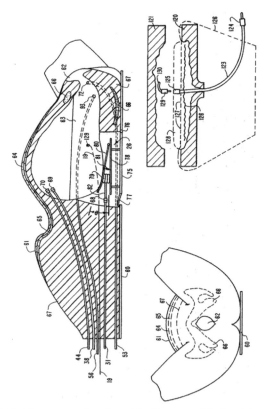

**Fig. 2.** Mechanical birthing system developed by Knapp and Eades. (*From* Knapp, Charles F. and Eades, George S., "Dynamic Childbirth Simulator for Teaching Maternity Patient Care" (1974). Biomedical Engineering Faculty Patents. 9. https://uknowledge.uky.edu/cbme_patents/9.)

Scientific, Miami, FL) (**Fig. 3**).[27] Noelle started the line of manikins used for high-fidelity obstetric simulation that are ubiquitous is simulation centers around the country today.

Although gynecologic simulation began similarly to obstetrics with pelvic models to teach contraception, menstrual cycle, and gynecologic problems, it shifted to teaching laparoscopic and other surgical skills as these technologies became more prominent.[28,29] After laparoscopy became recognized by the American Board of Obstetrics and Gynecology (ABOG) in 1971, the first laparoscopic training device for gynecologists was invented in 1985 by Semm,[30] a German gynecologist, and utilized a clear cover to allow learners to see their movements. In the decades that followed, research emerged that these box trainers improved surgical skills in the operating room, and laparoscopy simulation became the standard in residency training programs.[31–34] As technology has improved, so have the available simulation modalities.[35] Even today's learners in obstetrics and gynecology, however, still benefit from basic box trainers.[36]

## CURRENT TECHNOLOGY IN SIMULATION

Today, most advancing simulation models rely heavily of computer programs developed to mimic real-life obstetrics as closely as possible. The newest high-fidelity simulator from Gaumard, Victoria, includes programmable features ranging as simple as normal vaginal birth to eclamptic seizure and maternal code (**Fig. 4**). The lifelike qualities of the manikin include a weight of 77 kgs, which helps participants with realism during a code simulation, and blinking and breathing at rest. The accompanying computer system has a fetal heart rate tracing system that displays Doppler heart tones and tocometry as well as blood pressure, oxygenation, and pulse obtained through lifelike monitors placed on the manikin. There also is an infant simulator with programmable vital signs and ability to simulate an infant code. Although this technology is impressive, the cost of the manikin is more than $100,000 and typically requires a trained operator to perform the functions, discussed previously. For simulation programs that are just beginning or those that are established but lack substantial funding for high-fidelity simulators, there are other options that are cheaper.

Operative Experience (North East, MD), for example, has a Cesarean section model featuring a torso that simulates the multiple layers encountered when performing a Cesarean section as well as replicable uteri and babies to practice difficult fetal extractions (**Fig. 5**). Their models do not have electronic components but instead feature realistic tissue textures to aid with identifying various abdominal wall structures and, as such, are appreciably less expensive and easier to transport. This may be desirable

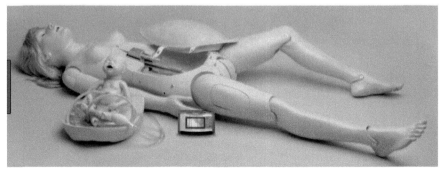

**Fig. 3.** Noelle: full patient manikin with a motorized mechanism for pushing. (*Courtesy of Gaumard Scientific, Miami, FL; with permission.*)

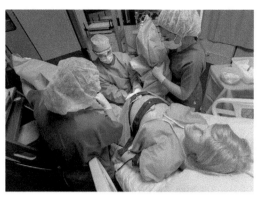

**Fig. 4.** Victoria obstetric simulator for Gaumard Scientific. (*Courtesy of* Gaumard Scientific, Miami, FL; with permission.)

for under-resourced countries as well, and Operative Experience has received funding to participate in an international effort to reduce maternal mortality from obstructed labor.[37] Another example of a focused device is the PROMPT birthing simulator (Laerdal Medical, Stavanger, Norway), which encompasses a pelvis and infant manikin that simulate shoulder dystocia (**Fig. 6**). Unique to this device is software that allows measurement of force applied to the baby. This allows real-time assessment of the pressure required to relieve a shoulder dystocia and pressures high enough to cause brachial plexus injury. A third example is the MamaNatalie hybrid simulator from Laerdal Medical (**Fig. 7**). This simulator features a wearable uterus with a reservoir basin to hold fake blood and allow for simulation of postpartum hemorrhage with predetermined blood loss. The patient, played by an actor, wears the device and controls the speed of bleeding, which is characteristic of a hybrid model.

Other areas of obstetric care currently simulated include procedures that are less commonly encountered or indicated in today's practice, such as forceps-assisted vaginal delivery and fourth-degree laceration repair. Modified beef tongue models have been used to simulate fourth-degree laceration repair and are an example of a low-cost, effective means of simulating.[38] And simulation of forceps-assisted vaginal delivery using a SimMom (Laerdal Medical; Stavanger, Norway) manikin (another full-body birthing simulator similar to Victoria obstetric simulator for Gaumard Scientific) have been shown to decrease rates of third-degree and fourth-degree lacerations in

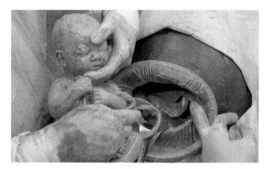

**Fig. 5.** Operative Experience's difficult fetal extraction simulator. (*Courtesy of* Operative Experience, North East, MD; with permission.)

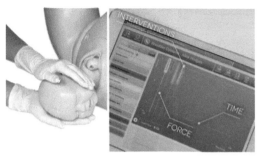

**Fig. 6.** PROMPT Flex—advanced birth simulator with real-time force detection. Left panel is birthing simulator. Right panel is graphic display of force in real-time. (*Courtesy of* Laerdal Medical, Stavanger, Norway; with permission.)

clinical practice.[39] There also are simulators available for obstetric subspecialties. In maternal-fetal medicine, chorionic villus sampling, amniocentesis, percutaneous umbilical blood sampling, and fetal surgery all have available simulation models. Sonography is another field with a wide array of available simulation programs to teach both novice sonographers and advanced skills depending on the program. VR has been a promising modality for sonography because self-guided learning is preferred.[40]

Current gynecology simulation technology also encompasses VR trainers that afford high fidelity and haptic feedback. LapMentor (3D Systems, Littleton, Colorado) is an example of one of these VR programs with tutorials on laparoscopic hysterectomy (**Fig. 8**).[35] VR offers the advantage of full-immersion medical simulation with all the distractions of a virtual team, equipment, and patient without requiring other participants to be present. This is ideal for self-directed learning but the lack of real-time human feedback, especially from an experienced surgeon, should not be overlooked because novice surgeons have been shown to perform fewer errors with fewer repetitions when instructed by an expert surgeon.[41,42]

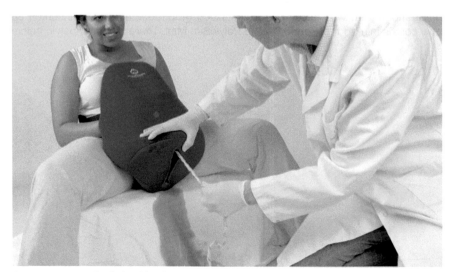

**Fig. 7.** MamaNatalie hybrid birth simulator. (*Courtesy of* Laerdal Medical, Stavanger, Norway; with permission.)

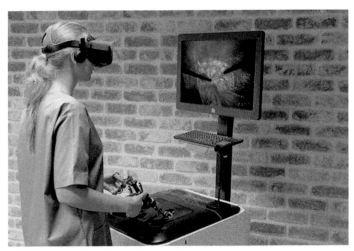

**Fig. 8.** LAP Mentor simulator from 3D Systems using VR. (*Courtesy of* 3D Systems, Littleton, CO; with permission.)

For those wanting practice in a simulated operating room without VR, porcine and ovine models have been studied for robotic hysterectomy and human cadavers have long been used for a variety of laparoscopic and open procedures.[43–46] Some physicians, including learners, may express ethical concerns with using animal or cadaveric models. As an alternative, SynDaver cadaver (SynDaver, Tampa Bay, Florida) offers a synthetic cadaver with tissue layers, blood vessels, and nerves to mimic an actual cadaver (**Fig. 9**). Each cadaver, however, is approximately $60,000, which may be cost-prohibitive for many training programs or hospital systems.[35]

Other areas of simulators currently available in gynecology include first-trimester and second-trimester surgical abortion as well as contraceptive device insertion with pelvic models.[47–50] The PelvicSim (VirtaMed, Zurich, Switzerland) is a portable pelvis model that was designed for simulation of intrauterine system insertion and now comes in a portable option called PelvicSim Mini. There are other pelvic trainers

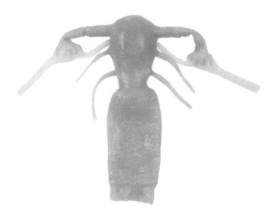

**Fig. 9.** SynDaver synthetic cadaver-like uterus. (Product of SynDaver, courtesy of Tech-Labs, Tech-Labs.com, Katy, TX; with permission.)

as well, with Limbs & Things (Bristol, United Kingdom) offering an example of one that comes with 7 different uterine models to diagnose various uterine pathology. Finally, some innovators in the field of simulation have developed a papaya model to train residents on manual vacuum aspiration.[51]

## CURRENT EVIDENCE FOR SIMULATION

Although it is clear that the simulation industry is large and ubiquitous, evidence in the literature supporting its use in clinical practice is more nuanced. An understanding of the available evidence to support the use of simulation is imperative for clinicians and educators in the health care field.

Research in simulation often is divided into Kirkpatrick's 4 levels of evaluation model because the purpose of simulation is to teach learners and assess how that learning impacted the organization.[52] The levels are fairly straightforward: level 1 assesses how participants felt after the training (confidence scores and surveys), level 2 assesses knowledge or skill performance (tests and assessment of skills), level 3 assesses if workplace behavior changed (auditing in clinical sites), and, finally, level 4 assesses organizational benefits (patient outcomes). Higher levels require more work from the simulationist but yield more coveted results. That being said, sometimes level 1 and level 2 outcomes are sufficient to answer the question being asked. For example, DeStephano and colleagues[13] studied if high-fidelity simulation (Noelle birth simulator) was superior to a hybrid birth simulator (MamaNatalie) for teaching medical students vaginal delivery. They assessed students' confidence (level 1) and performance of delivery skills (level 2) and found no difference in skill performance. Surprisingly, students were more confident following the simulation with a hybrid simulator. This has important implications for validating hybrid simulators as an effective teaching tool but also acknowledging that stage of training for the learner may have an impact on the type of simulator used.

Still, the most desired research outcomes are those that demonstrate improved patient outcomes because this is the utmost goal of simulation. The first area of obstetric simulation to demonstrate improved outcomes was in management of shoulder dystocia.[53] In 2008, Draycott and colleagues[53] reported outcomes from the SaFE (Simulation and Fire-drill Evaluation) trial, which followed several hospitals in the United Kingdom as they underwent training in advanced maneuvers and team communication surrounding a shoulder dystocia simulation. Following implementation, they found the usage of advanced maneuvers by providers increased (level 3 data). More importantly, they found a 4-fold reduction in number of brachial plexus injuries from the presimulation era to the postsimulation era, despite the rate of shoulder dystocia being consistent. This was significant as one of the first studies to demonstrate improved patient outcomes following simulation. In 2011, Inglis and colleagues[54] were able to demonstrate a 3-fold reduction in brachial plexus injury following implementation of shoulder dystocia simulation at their institution in New York.

Thus far, shoulder dystocia has been the most prolific area of research able to demonstrate improved patient outcomes. When looking at postpartum hemorrhage simulation, for example, prior literature has been able to demonstrate medication errors made by residents and underestimation of blood loss as well as improved communication skills, confidence and interdisciplinary relationships (levels 1 and 2), but there is a paucity of data regarding improved patient outcomes.[55–57] In a Norwegian study, the number of red blood cell transfusions decreased following mandatory interdisciplinary postpartum hemorrhage simulation, but the researchers cautioned that complex interactions involving several variables could confound the results.[58]

Nelissen and colleagues[59] were able to demonstrate a more robust outcome as they showed a 38% reduction in incidence of postpartum hemorrhage following implementation of a simulation program in Tanzania using MamaNatalie. Simulation research related to eclampsia has had less fruitful results. Ellis and Crofts,[60] from the SaFe trial, were able to show improved completion of checklist items, including administration of magnesium sulfate, and shorter time from seizure to magnesium delivery (level 3). Patient outcomes in the eclampsia simulation literature, however, are lacking.

Although patient outcome improvements are scarcer in the literature, improvements in teamwork and communication of multidisciplinary teams have been easier to demonstrate. In a systematic review of the obstetric literature for simulation and teamwork in 2010, Merien and colleagues[61] found 7 studies showing that communication and team performance were both improved by teamwork training. Phipps and colleagues[62] also found that communication and teamwork were closely linked when evaluating outcomes following implementation of a multidisciplinary team training program. Finally, multidisciplinary team training has demonstrated not only improvement in communication and teamwork, but also in safety culture.[2,63–65] Because communication errors are associated with a majority of sentinel events, it naturally follows that improving communication is beneficial for preventing medical errors and providing safer patient care.

For surgical simulation in gynecology, there is abundant evidence supporting laparoscopic simulation for teaching gynecologic surgeries.[31–36] As a result, the ABOG now requires Fundamentals of Laparoscopic Surgery (FLS) module completion in order to sit for written board examinations. FLS is a Web-based curriculum with a hands-on training and skills assessment component that ABOG describes as part of a broader initiative to incorporate simulation into training completed by obstetricians-gynecologists. In addition to teaching initial skill sets, Mannella and colleagues[66] compared task completion of junior residents versus senior residents and found both groups improved in technical skills. VR simulators also have demonstrated efficacy in teaching laparoscopic surgical skills.[67] Hart and colleagues[67] demonstrated improved surgical skills following laparoscopic salpingectomy, salpingotomy, and tubal clipping via a VR platform. As discussed previously, cadaveric dissection also has been shown to improve proficiency in surgical anatomy and is uniquely able to provide robotic, laparoscopic and open procedural experience.[46] All the modalities discussed previously (laparoscopic trainers, cadavers, and VR) have been shown to improve surgical skills.[68]

Outside of the operating room, office-based gynecology procedures also may be simulated effectively and recommended as part of American College of Obstetricians and Gynecologists (ACOG) Safety Certification in Outpatient Practice Excellence.[69] Espey and colleagues[70] created a curriculum for simulating office-based procedural emergency scenarios, including seizure, anaphylaxis, and hemorrhage, and were able to show improve confidence and performance (levels 1 and 2).

## FUTURE DIRECTIONS

Despite the lack of literature supporting improved patient outcomes, there has been universal acceptance of simulation as a staple on labor and delivery units by most national organizations. In 2012, ACOG released their "Quality patient care in labor and delivery: a call to action," which was endorsed by American Academy of Family Physicians; American Academy of Pediatrics; American College of Nurse-Midwives; American College of Osteopathic Obstetricians and Gynecologists; Association of Women's Health, Obstetrics, and Neonatal Nurses; and Society for Maternal-Fetal Medicine.[71] In this document, they recommend regular drills and simulations as well as debriefings and communication tools to provide safe, effective patient care. This closely aligns with the Alliance for Innovation on Maternal health (AIM) patient safety bundles because many of them recommend simulations and/or drills as part of improving maternal care. These safety bundles have been adopted by many states and are in various stages of implementation across the country in conjunction with initiatives by several other national organizations all with the goal of improving maternal care.[72]

More recently, the Joint Commission has released new requirements for hospital accreditation with the purpose of improving maternal safety from hemorrhage and severe hypertension/preeclampsia.[73] Standards PC.06.01.01 and PC.06.01.03 closely resemble the AIM bundles on hemorrhage and severe hypertension, respectively. As such, they require hospitals to conduct multidisciplinary drills in an effort to identify system issues as part of ongoing quality improvement and encourage the incorporation of disciplines found outside of labor and delivery to "test" these systems in the safe environment of simulation. As more safety bundles are implemented across the country, it is possible the list of simulation requirements for hospitals will continue to grow.

At a more local level, and no doubt as a reflection of pressure from national organizations, some hospitals now require simulation annually for physician privileges either for obstetric emergencies or skill demonstration for certain procedures. Some malpractice insurers also have joined this movement and are requiring documentation of participation in simulation prior to insuring the individual. Finally, the process for board certification maintenance for anesthesiologists now contains a simulation option, which lends itself to the question if the ABOG will follow suit.

Regardless of the path that future research in simulation and governing organizations takes, it is clear that simulation in obstetrics and gynecology is here to stay. Reduction in the medical work force to have more work-life balance, decreased indications for gynecologic surgeries and focus on restricting both resident duty hours and attending physician burnout calls for the availability to practice clinical scenarios outside of patient care to maintain proficiency. Simulation provides the perfect venue to fill the void of decreased clinical experience while easing fears from patients that they are being practiced on and assuring malpractice insurers and hospitals alike that physicians are well trained and prepared for any emergency. Lastly, the physician workforce is rapidly filling with the millennial generation who have been taught simulation throughout their matriculation and are more accepting of its use in medicine than older generations. For all of these reasons, simulation in obstetrics and gynecology will continue to grow in both scope and depth.

## CLINICS CARE POINTS

- Simulation is a vital tool to improve clinical skills and patient safety in both obstetrics and gynecology.
- High-fidelity, low-fidelity, and hybrid-fidelity simulation models all have proved beneficial.
- Implementing team-based shoulder dystocia training has been shown to decrease brachial plexus injuries.
- Team-based training in obstetrics has been shown to improve communication and team performance.
- Gynecologic surgery simulation has proven effective using simple constructs, such as box trainers, more realistic models, such as unembalmed cadavers, and more advanced technology using VR.

## REFERENCES

1. Kohn LT, Corrigan J, Donaldson MS. To Err is human: building a safer health system. Washington, DC: National Academies Press; 2000.
2. Siassakos D, Draycott T, Montague I, et al. Content analysis of team communication in an obstetric emergency scenario. J Obstet Gynaecol 2009;29:499–503.
3. Robertson B, Schumacher L, Gosman G, et al. Simulation-based crisis team training for multidisciplinary obstetric providers. Simul Healthc 2009;4(2):77–83.
4. Aggarwal R, Mytton OT, Derbrew M, et al. Training and simulation for patient safety. BMJ Qual Saf 2010;19:i34–43.
5. Al-Elq AH. Simulation-based medical teaching and learning. J Fam Community Med 2010;17(1):35–40.
6. Ahmed RA, Frey J, Gardner AK, et al. Characteristics and core curricular elements of medical simulation fellowships in North America. J Grad Med Educ 2016;8(2):252–5.
7. Owen H, Pelosi MA. A historical examination of the budin-pinard phantom: what can contemporary obstetrics education learn from simulators of the past? Acad Med 2013;88(5):652–6.
8. Thomas MP. The role of simulation in the development of technical competence during surgical training: a literature review. Int J Med Educ 2013;4:48–58.
9. Good M, Gravenstein J. Anesthesia simulators and training devices. Int Anesthesiol Clin 1989;27:161–6.
10. Cooper J, Taqueti VR. A brief history of the development of mannequin simulators for clinical education and training. Qual Saf Health Care 2004;13:i11–8.
11. Chiniara G, Cole G, Brisbin K, et al, Canadian Network For Simulation In Healthcare, Guidelines Working Group. Simulation in healthcare: a taxonomy and a conceptual framework for instructional design and media selection. Med Teach 2013; 35(8):e1380–95.
12. Munshi F, Lababidi H, Alyousef S. Low- versus high-fidelity simulations in teaching and assessing clinical skills. J Taibah Univ Med Sci 2015;10(1):12–5.
13. DeStephano CC, Chou B, Patel S, et al. A randomized controlled trial of birth simulation for medical students. Am J Obstet Gynecol 2015;213:91.e1–7.
14. Taekman JM, Shelley K. Virtual environments in healthcare: immersion, disruption, and flow. Int Anesthesiol Clin 2010;48(3):101–21.
15. Chmil JV. Prebriefing in simulation-based learning experiences. Nurse Educ 2016;41(2):64–5.
16. Copyright 2004-2020 Center for Medical Simulation, Boston, Massachusetts, USA. Available at: www.harvardmedsim.org info@havardmedsim.org. Accessed January 1, 2021.
17. Fanning RM, Gaba DM. The role of debriefing in simulation-based learning. Simul Healthc 2007;2(2):115–25.
18. Rudolph JW, Simon R, Dufresne RL, et al. There's no such thing as "nonjudgmental" debriefing: a theory and method for debriefing with good judgment. Simul Healthc 2006;1(1):49–55.
19. Eppich W, Cheng A. Promoting excellence and reflective learning in simulation (PEARLS). Simul Healthc 2015;10(2):106–15.
20. Cody LF. Breeding Scottish obstetrics in Dr. Smellie's London. In: Birthing a nation: sex, science and the conception of eighteenth century Britons. New York: Oxford University Press; 2005. p. 152–97.
21. Buck GH. Development of simulators in medical education. Gesnerus 1991; 48:7–28.

22. Wilson A. A new synthesis: William Smellie. In: The making of man-midwifery: childbirth in England 1660–1770. London: University College London Press; 1995. p. 123–33.
23. Gelbart NR. The King's midwife: a history and mystery of Madame du Coudray. Los Angeles, CA: University of California Press; 1998.
24. Schultes medacta GmbH & Co. Lehrmodelle KG. Available at: http://www. schultes-medacta.de/index.html. Accessed January 1, 2021.
25. Knapp CF, Eades GS. Dynamic childbirth simulator for teaching maternity patient care. Biomed Eng Fac Patents 1974;9.
26. Abrahamson S, Denson JS, Wolf RM. Effectiveness of a simulator in training anesthesiology residents. The J Med Education 1969;44(6):515–9.
27. Gaumard Scientific Co., Inc. Miami, FL. (1998. Inventors: Eggert JS (Miami, FL), Eggert MS (Birmingham, MD) and Vallejo P (Miami, FL). Available at: https://www. gaumard.com/products/obstetrics/noelle. Accessed January 1, 2021.
28. Gardner R, Raemer DB. Simulation in obstetrics and gynecology. Obstet Gynecol Clin North Am 2008;35:97–127.
29. Semm K. Operative pelviscopy. Br Med Bull 1986;42:284–95.
30. Semm K. [Pelvi-trainer, a training device in operative pelviscopy for teaching endoscopic ligation and suture technics]. Geburtshilfe Fraueheilkd 1986;46: 60–2 [in German].
31. Scott DJ, Bergen PC, Rege RV, et al. Laparoscopic training on bench models: better and more cost effective than operating room experience? J Am Coll Surg 2000;191:272–83.
32. Dawe SR, Pena GN, Windsor JA, et al. Systematic review of skills transfer after surgical simulation-based training. Br J Surg 2014;101:1063–76.
33. Nagendran M, Toon CD, Davidson BR, et al. Laparoscopic surgical box model training for surgical trainees with no prior laparoscopic experience. Cochrane Database Syst Rev 2014;1:Cd010479.
34. Gurusamy KS, Nagendran M, Toon CD, et al. Laparoscopic surgical box model training for surgical trainees with limited prior laparoscopic experience. Cochrane Database Syst Rev 2014;3:Cd010478.
35. Wohlrab K, Jelovsek JE, Myers D. Incorporating simulation into gynecologic surgical training. Am J Obstet Gynecol 2017;217(5):522–6.
36. Wilson E, Janssens S, McLindon LA, et al. Improved laparoscopic skills in gynaecology trainees following a simulation-training program using take-home box trainers. Aust N Z J Obstet Gynaecol 2019;59:110–6.
37. Available at: https://operativeexperience.com/clients-and-partners/. Accessed January 1, 2021.
38. Illston JD, Ballard AC, Ellington DR, et al. Modified beef tongue model for fourth-degree laceration repair simulation. Obstet Gynecol 2017;129:491–6.
39. Gossett DR, Gilchrist-Scott D, Wayne DB, et al. Simulation training for forceps-assisted vaginal delivery and rates of maternal perineal trauma. Obstet Gynecol 2016;128:429–35.
40. Burden C, Preshaw J, White P, et al. Validation of virtual reality simulation for obstetric ultrasonography: a prospective cross-sectional study. Simul Healthc 2012; 7(5):269–73.
41. Van Sickle KR, Gallagher AG, Smith CD. The effect of escalating feedback on the acquisition of psychomotor skills for laparoscopy. Surg Endosc 2007;21:220–4.
42. Trehan A, Bartnett-Vanes A, Carty MJ, et al. The impact of feedback of intraoperative technical performance in surgery: a systematic review. BMJ Open 2015;5: e006759.

43. Hoffman MS. Simulation of robotic hysterectomy utilizing the porcine model. Am J Obstet Gynecol 2012;206(6):523.e1–2.
44. Alshiek J, Bar-El L, Shobeiri S. Vaginal Robotic Supracervical Hysterectomy in an Ovine Animal Model: The Proof of Concept. Open J Obstet Gynecol 2019;9: 1114–29.
45. Lim CP, Roberts M, Chalhoub T, et al. Cadaveric surgery in core gynaecology training: a feasibility study [published correction appears in Gynecol Surg. 2018;15(1):5]. Gynecol Surg 2018;15(1):4.
46. Corton MM, Wai CY, Vakili B, et al. A comprehensive pelvic dissection course improves obstetrics and gynecology resident proficiency in surgical anatomy. Am J Obstet Gynecol 2003;189(3):647–51.
47. Storey A, White K, Treder K, et al. First-Trimester Abortion Complications: Simulation Cases for OB/GYN Residents in Sepsis and Hemorrhage. MedEdPORTAL 2020;16:10995.
48. Baldwin MK, Chor J, Chen BA, et al. Comparison of 3 dilation and evacuation technical skills models. J Grad Med Educ 2013;5(4):662–4.
49. Dodge LE, Hacker MR, Averbach SH, et al. Assessment of a high-fidelity mobile simulator for intrauterine contraception training in ambulatory reproductive health centres. J Eur CME 2016;5(1):30416.
50. Creinin MD, Kaunitz AM, Darney PD, et al. The US etonogestrel implant mandatory clinical training and active monitoring programs: 6-year experience. Contraception 2017;95(2):205–10.
51. Paul M, Nobel K. Papaya: a simulation model for training in uterine aspiration. Fam Med 2005;37(4):242–4.
52. Bewley WL, O'Neil HF. Evaluation of medical simulations. Mil Med 2013;178(10 Suppl):64–75.
53. Draycott TJ, Crofts JF, Ash JP, et al. Improving neonatal outcome through practical shoulder dystocia training. Obstet Gynecol 2008;112(1):14–20.
54. Inglis SR, Feier N, Chetiyaar JB, et al. Effects of shoulder dystocia training on the incidence of brachial plexus injury. Am J Obstet Gynecol 2011;204(4):322.e1–6.
55. Deering SH, Chinn M, Hodor J, et al. Use of a postpartum hemorrhage simulator for instruction and evaluation of residents. J Grad Med Educ 2009;1(2):260–3.
56. Reynolds A, Ayres-de-Campos D, Bastos L, et al. Impact of labor and delivery simulation classes in undergraduate medical learning. Med Educ Online 2008; 13:14.
57. Maslovitz S, Barkai G, Lessing JB, et al. Improved accuracy of postpartum blood loss estimation as assessed by simulation. Acta Obstet Gynecol Scand 2008; 87(9):929–34.
58. Egenberg S, Oian P, Bru LE, et al. Can inter-profressional simulation training influence the frequency of blood transfusions after birth? Acta Obstet Gynecol Scand 2015;94:316–23.
59. Nelissen E, Ersdal H, Mduma E, et al. Clinical performance and patient outcome after simulation-based training in prevention and management of postpartum haemorrhage: an educational intervention study in a low-resource setting. BMC Pregnancy Childbirth 2017;17:301.
60. Ellis D, Crofts JF, Hunt LP, et al. Hospital, simulation center, and teamwork training for eclampsia management: a randomized controlled trial. Obstet Gynecol 2008; 111(3):723–31.
61. Merien AER, van de Ven J, Mol BW, et al. Multidisciplinary team training in a simulation setting for acute obstetric emergencies. Obstet Gynecol 2010;115: 1021–31.

62. Phipps MG, Lindquist DG, McConaughey E, et al. Outcomes from a labor and delivery team training program with simulation component. Am J Obstet Gynecol 2012;206:3–9.
63. Kirschbaum KA, Rask JP, Brennan M, et al. Improved climate, culture, and communication through multidisciplinary training and instruction. Am J Obstet Gynecol 2012;207:200.e1–7.
64. Siassakos D, Bristowe K, Draycott TJ, et al. Clinical efficiency in a simulated emergency and relationship to team behaviours: a multisite cross-sectional study. BJOG 2011;118:596–607.
65. Gardner R, Walzer TB, Simon R, et al. Obstetric simulation as a risk control strategy: course design and evaluation. Simul Healthc 2008;3(2):119–27.
66. Mannella P, Malacarne E, Giannini A, et al. Simulation as tool for evaluating and improving technical skills in laparoscopic gynecological surgery. BMC Surg 2019;19:146.
67. Hart R, Doherty DA, Karthigasu K, et al. The value of virtual reality–simulator training in the development of laparoscopic surgical skills. J Minim Invasive Gynecol 2006;13(2):126–33.
68. Thomas MP. The role of simulation in the development of technical competence during surgical training: a literature review. Int J Med Educ 2013;4:48–58.
69. Urman RD, Punwani N, Bombaugh M, et al. Safety considerations for office-based obstetric and gynecologic procedures. Rev Obstet Gynecol 2013;6(1): e8–14.
70. Espey E, Baty G, Rask J, et al. Emergency in the clinic: a simulation curriculum to improve outpatient safety. Am J Obstet Gynecol 2017;217(6):699.e1–13.
71. Lawrence HC, Copel JA, O'Keeffe DF, et al. Quality patient care in labor and delivery: a call to action. Am J Obstet Gynecol 2012;207:147–8.
72. Combs CA, Davidson C, Einerson BD, et al. SMFM special statement: who's who in patient safety and quality for maternal healthcare in the United States. Am J Obstet Gynecol 2020;223(1):B2–15.
73. Available at: https://www.jointcommission.org/standards/r3-report/r3-report-issue-24-pc-standards-for-maternal-safety/. Accessed January 1, 2021.

# The Current and Future States of Screening in Gynecologic Cancers

Jessica Lee, MD[a],*, Navya Nair, MD, MPH[b]

## KEYWORDS

- Cervical cancer • Endometrial cancer • Genetics • Gynecologic cancer • HPV
- Screening • Ovarian cancer • Prevention

## KEY POINTS

- Cervical cancer is the only gynecologic cancer with an effective screening test at this time.
- There is a great need for screening strategies in other gynecologic malignancies, especially ovarian cancer and type II endometrial cancers, which behave aggressively and have an overall poor prognosis.
- The future of gynecologic cancer screening will include more patient-centric, biomarker-driven screening modalities.

## INTRODUCTION

Gynecologic cancers account for significant morbidity and mortality in the United States and the world. These cancers consist of ovarian, fallopian tube, primary peritoneal, uterine, cervical, vulvar, and vaginal cancers, and represent approximately 10% to 15% of cancers in women. In 2020, it was estimated that 113,520 cases of gynecologic cancers would be diagnosed among US women and contribute to 33,620 deaths.[1] Advancements in early detection methods and identification of high-risk cohorts have reduced the risk of some of these malignancies over the last few decades. This article reviews current and up-and-coming screening strategies for the prevention and early detection of gynecologic malignancies.

[a] Division of Gynecologic Oncology, Department of Obstetrics & Gynecology, UT Southwestern Medical Center, 5323 Harry Hines Boulevard, G6. 224, Dallas, TX 75390, USA; [b] Division of Gynecologic Oncology, Department of Obstetrics & Gynecology, LSU Health Sciences Center – New Orleans, 1542 Tulane Avenue, 5th Floor, New Orleans, LA 70112, USA
* Corresponding author.
E-mail address: jessica2.lee@utsouthwestern.edu

Obstet Gynecol Clin N Am 48 (2021) 705–722
https://doi.org/10.1016/j.ogc.2021.06.001
0889-8545/21/© 2021 Elsevier Inc. All rights reserved.

obgyn.theclinics.com

## UTERINE CANCER

Uterine cancer is the most common gynecologic malignancy in the United States, with 65,620 new cases and 12,590 deaths estimated for 2020.[1] Rates of uterine cancer are increasing and, by 2030, it is projected to surpass colon cancer to become the third most common cancer among women.[2]

Endometrial cancer is classified into 2 broad subtypes: type I, which comprises 80% to 90% of endometrial cancers, and the less common type II. Type I carcinomas are of low histologic grade, are detected at early stages, and generally offer a favorable prognosis. They are typically associated with exposure to unopposed estrogen and preceded by endometrial intraepithelial neoplasia (EIN). Type II carcinomas comprise high-grade carcinomas, including grade 3 endometrioid, serous, clear cell, carcinosarcomas, and undifferentiated histologies. They tend to follow an aggressive clinical course, are more often diagnosed at advanced stages, and have a poorer prognosis than type I carcinomas. The precursor lesion for type II carcinomas is endometrial intraepithelial carcinoma, arising from an atrophic endometrium.[3]

Uterine sarcomas are a group of rare but aggressive uterine malignancies arising from the myometrium, accounting for only 1% of gynecologic cancers and 7% to 9% of all uterine cancers.[4,5] There are no effective screening mechanisms for uterine sarcomas at this time.

### Prevention of Endometrial Cancer in the General Population

Educating women about the early signs of endometrial cancer and its association with obesity would likely contribute to earlier detection.[6,7] Bariatric surgery to effect weight loss has shown decreased incidence of endometrial cancer as well as mortality associated with endometrial cancer.[8]

The use of combined oral contraceptive pills and progestin-based contraceptives has been shown to decrease the risk of endometrial cancer. The Norwegian Women and Cancer study showed that the levonorgestrel intrauterine device (IUD) reduced the endometrial cancer risk by 78%.[9] The prospective Progesterone Therapy for Endometrial Cancer (PROTEC) trial showed that the levonorgestrel IUD inserted in women with a body mass index (BMI) greater than 40 was well tolerated, improved bleeding patterns, and changed endometrial morphology. The study concluded that the IUD could provide a strategy for a prevention trial.[10]

### Increased Risk of Endometrial Cancer: Unopposed Estrogen

The most significant risk factor is exposure to unopposed estrogens, which cause proliferative changes in the endometrium. Persistent proliferative endometrium can then become hyperplastic and ultimately carcinomatous.[11] Obesity is the strongest risk factor for type I endometrial cancer and EIN. Women with BMIs of 40 or greater have an almost 10-fold higher lifetime risk of endometrial cancer compared with women of normal weight.[12] An estimated 30% to 40% of all endometrial cancers are directly attributable to obesity.[13] Dysregulation of adipocytokine production and inflammation, hyperinsulinemia, and sex-steroid hormones are hypothesized to underlie the adiposity-endometrial cancer link.[14] Polycystic ovarian syndrome also confers increased risk.[15]

Tamoxifen is a selective estrogen receptor modulator used for the treatment and prevention of estrogen receptor–positive breast cancer that acts as an estrogen agonist on the endometrium. The National Surgical Adjuvant Breast and Bowel Project trial reported a 2.2-fold to 2.3-fold increased risk of endometrial cancer in patients with breast cancer on tamoxifen for 5 years.[16]

### Increased Risk of Endometrial Cancer: Genetic Variants

Approximately 3% to 5% of endometrial cancers are caused by an inherited variant. Lynch syndrome is the most common inherited cancer predisposition syndrome that increases the lifetime risk of developing endometrial cancer. Lynch syndrome is caused by autosomal dominant variants in the *MLH1*, *MSH2*, *MSH6*, and *PMS2* genes or a deletion in the *EPCAM* gene. The cumulative incidence of endometrial cancer by the age of 80 years ranges from 13% to 54% based on the specific genetic variant.[17]

### Increased Risk of Poor Prognosis Associated with Endometrial Cancer: Black Race

Black women in the United States are disproportionately affected by the burden of endometrial cancer. They are more likely to be diagnosed at higher stages and have poorer survival at every stage of disease after controlling for other factors.[18] Black women are less likely to have guideline-adherent evaluation of postmenopausal bleeding, which is the most common presenting symptom of endometrial cancer.[19] The American College of Obstetricians and Gynecologists (ACOG) recommends evaluation of any postmenopausal bleeding with transvaginal ultrasonography (TVUS) and subsequent endometrial biopsy if the endometrial thickness is found to be greater than 4 mm on TVUS. This algorithm, which is the current standard of care, was recently evaluated among a simulated cohort of black women and was found to miss half of all endometrial cancers in this population.[20] Decreased effectiveness of ACOG's algorithm in black women may contribute to this population being diagnosed with endometrial cancer at higher stages. Acknowledging and addressing racial disparities and devising strategies that work in all patient populations is critical in mitigating the undue endometrial cancer disease burden among black women in the United States.

### Screening for Low-Risk Individuals

Nearly 75% of endometrial cancers are detected at an early stage, and 5-year survival rates exceed 90%.[21] Approximately 9% of women with postmenopausal bleeding were found to have endometrial cancer.[22] Because more than 90% of women are symptomatic at the time of early-stage endometrial cancer, there are no recommendations for screening in low-risk, asymptomatic women.[23]

### Screening for Intermediate-Risk Individuals

There are no current recommendations for screening in women with predisposing risk factors, including morbid obesity, unopposed estrogen exposure, or tamoxifen use. These women should be counseled on their increased risk of endometrial cancer and educated on warning symptoms to monitor. In a study of asymptomatic women using tamoxifen, screening for endometrial cancer with routine TVUS, endometrial biopsy, or both has not been shown to be effective.[24–26]

### Screening for High-Risk Individuals

Endometrial cancer screening has not been shown to be beneficial in high-risk women with Lynch syndrome. Similar to low-risk or intermediate-risk women, endometrial cancer can often be detected at an early stage based on symptoms, and, therefore, high-risk women should be educated on the importance of prompt reporting and evaluation of any abnormal uterine or postmenopausal bleeding. Screening with endometrial biopsies every 1 to 2 years from age 30 to 35 years has been proposed because endometrial biopsies are highly sensitive and specific as a diagnostic procedure.

### Future Directions in Endometrial Cancer Screening

Since the 1970s, cancer survival has improved for all of the most common cancers, except for endometrial cancer.[27] Stagnant survival rates largely reflect not only a need for new therapeutics but also a paucity of innovative prevention and screening strategies.

Although endometrial biopsies have high sensitivity and specificity, they are invasive and often uncomfortable. New advances allow the detection of molecular alterations with a high sensitivity, compared with traditional methods. Urine is being studied to identify biomarkers, either excreted by the kidneys or shed from the uterus (**Fig. 1**). Endometrial cancer cells may also be isolated from urine, especially in women with bleeding symptoms, by cytology, or by use of single-cell technology. Urinary cell-free circulating tumor DNA (ctDNA) may be renally excreted or may be shed from the uterus following breakdown of malignant or premalignant cells contaminating urinary flow.[28] Vaginally collected biospecimens have also been studied in the evaluation of endometrial cancer. Women self-placed an intravaginal tampon that was retained in the vagina for 30 minutes before their hysterectomies. Endometrial cancer–specific DNA methylation markers were isolated in the vaginal samples from the tampons. Women diagnosed with endometrial cancer were found to have higher levels of DNA methylation markers compared with control samples.[29]

Methods on cervical sampling either at the time of Pap test or with other technologies to detect endometrial cancer have been evaluated in various proof-of-concept studies (**Fig. 2**). Cervicovaginal levels of cancer antigen 125 (CA-125) were assessed in women diagnosed with either endometrial cancer or EIN. The CA-125 levels were found to be increased but overall had low specificity and positive predictive value.[30]

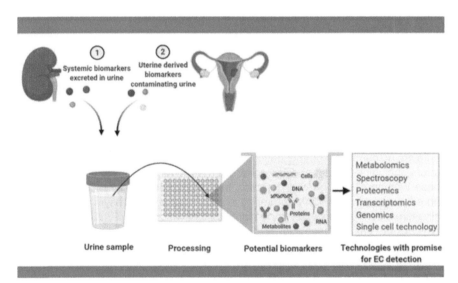

**Fig. 1.** Urinary biomarkers may be renally excreted or may be shed from the uterus following breakdown of malignant or premalignant cells contaminating urinary flow. These biomarkers can then be studied with cytology, spectroscopy, metabolomics, transcriptomics, and proteomics. EC, endometrial cancer. (*From* Njoku K, Chiasserini D, Jones ER, et al. Urinary Biomarkers and Their Potential for the Non-Invasive Detection of Endometrial Cancer. Front Oncol. 2020;10:559016. Published 2020 Nov 3. https://doi.org/10.3389/fonc.2020. 559016, Creative Commons Attribution License (CC BY).)

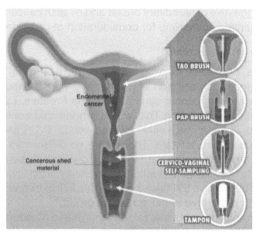

**Fig. 2.** Various minimally invasive sampling methods have been proposed to detect preinvasive or invasive endometrial cancer. The sampling methods are listed in increasing degree of invasiveness (*upward arrow*). (*From* Costas L, Frias-Gomez J, Guardiola M, et al. New perspectives on screening and early detection of endometrial cancer. Int J Cancer. 2019;145(12):3194-3206. https://doi.org/10.1002/ijc.32514; with permission.)

Activity of total proprotein convertases, a family of serine proteases, has been found to be increased in endocervical swabs and uterine lavages in women with endometrial cancer compared with controls.[31] Similar to the ovarian cancer studies, various studies on Pap tests have collected fluid to detect malignant or premalignant cells, and to perform epigenetic and genetic studies, which can be performed via polymerase chain reaction (PCR)–based tests.[32,33] Genomic analysis of driver mutations collected via uterine lavage have been able to identify women with endometrial cancer.[34]

## OVARIAN CANCER

In 2020, it is estimated that there will be 21,750 new cases of ovarian cancer diagnosed in the United States, and, despite advances of treatment, an estimated 13,940 women will die of this disease.[1] Although a woman's risk of developing ovarian cancer during her lifetime is approximately 1 in 78, it is the deadliest of all gynecologic cancers. Ovarian cancer is the fifth leading cause of cancer deaths among women in the United States.[35] Research in developing screening and early detection strategies has been ongoing to prevent invasive cancer or to diagnosis ovarian cancer in its early stages to reduce its high mortality.

### Increased Risk of Ovarian Cancer: Genetic Variants

Inherited variants account for approximately 15% to 25% of invasive ovarian cancers.[36,37] Most hereditary ovarian cancers are caused by variants in the *BRCA1* and *BRCA2* genes, which confer a lifetime ovarian cancer risk of 44% and 17%, respectively.[38] Other genetic variants associated with inherited ovarian cancer include *BRIP1*, *PALB2*, *RAD51C*, *RAD15D*, and Lynch syndrome genes (*MLH1*, *MSH2*, *MSH6*, *PMS2*, and *EPCAM*).[36] It is strongly recommended by multiple professional organizations, including the Society of Gynecologic Oncology (SGO), for individuals with family histories suggestive of hereditary breast and ovarian cancer or Lynch syndrome to be referred to genetic counseling for consideration of germline genetic testing.

### Screening for Low-Risk Individuals

The United States Preventive Services Task Force (USPSTF) has recommended against ovarian cancer screening in asymptomatic women who are not known to have a high-risk hereditary cancer syndrome.[39] The Prostate, Lung, Colorectal and Ovarian (PLCO) Cancer Screening Trial was a randomized controlled trial in which women aged 55 to 74 years were either offered annual TVUS and serum CA-125 or continued with routine medical care. There were no differences in the incidence of ovarian cancer or the cancer stage at time of diagnosis between two groups. There was no statistically significant reduction in mortality from ovarian cancer in the screened cohort. There was a 5% false-positive rate in this trial, which led to more oophorectomies being performed in the screening group.[40]

The largest randomized control trial to date, the United Kingdom Collaborative Trial of Ovarian Cancer Screening (UKCTOCS) trial, enrolled more than 200,000 asymptomatic women aged 50 to 74 years. The women were divided into 3 groups: (1) no screening, (2) multimodal screening with annual serum CA-125 interpreted with the Risk of Ovarian Cancer Algorithm (ROCA) and follow-up TVUS if the CA-125 proved to be abnormal, and (3) annual TVUS. There were no differences in the incidence of ovarian cancer among the 3 groups, but there were women diagnosed with more low-volume disease in the multimodal group compared with the no-screening group. Despite the potential stage shift, there was no overall improvement seen in mortality with multimodal screening.[41]

Based on the current data, the USPSTF has concluded that ovarian cancer screening in low-risk women does not reduce ovarian cancer mortality, and it can result in harm from false-positive tests leading to unnecessary surgeries in women without cancer.[39]

### Screening for High-Risk Individuals

No screening strategy has been shown to definitively improve detection of early-stage ovarian cancer in high-risk women to improve survival rates. The National Comprehensive Cancer Network (NCCN) currently suggests TVUS with CA-125 for ovarian cancer screening with women starting at 30 to 35 years, although there is uncertain benefit.[42] Therefore, the standard of care is a risk-reducing bilateral salpingo-oophorectomy (RRSO) at age 35 to 45 years, following completion of childbearing. Prospective and observational studies have shown an 80% to 85% reduction in ovarian cancer risk in BRCA carriers following RRSO and a 77% reduction in all-cause mortality.[43,44]

Studies have evaluated various screening modalities in high-risk populations. In the United Kingdom Familial Ovarian Cancer Screening Study (UK FOCSS), 4348 women with an overall lifetime risk of at least 10% were identified. They underwent ovarian cancer screening with pelvic sonograms and serum CA-125 every 4 months, interpreted using ROCA. Out of the 4348 women, 19 patients were diagnosed with invasive ovarian cancer, of whom 13 were detected as a result of the screening protocol. More than half of the women diagnosed with cancer were of early stage (stage I to II) at time of diagnosis, showing a stage shift. Sensitivity, positive predictive value, and negative predictive value of the screening protocol for detecting ovarian cancer within 1 year were 94.7%, 10.8%, and 100%, respectively.[45]

Another trial investigated 3692 women with strong breast or ovarian cancer family histories or BRCA1/2 variants to assess a screening protocol involving serial serum CA-125 levels every 3 months, interpreted using ROCA, possibly triggering follow-up TVUS. This study identified 6 incidental ovarian cancers, of which 50% were early stage.[46]

These studies suggest that screening with serial CA-125 levels with TVUS is an option for high-risk women and showed high sensitivity and significant shift toward early stages. However, neither study was able to show improved survival with the screening protocol in these high-risk women. Therefore, RRSO remains the current standard of care for ovarian cancer risk management. NCCN recommends that this occur by age 35 to 40 years in women with *BRCA1/2*, although consideration could be made to delay until age 40 to 45 years in *BRCA2*. For women with *BRIP1*, *RAD51C*, and *RAD51D* variants, consideration for RRSO could be made at age 45 to 50 years. There are not yet guidelines for RRSO for women with *PALB2* variants[42] (**Table 1**).

### Future Directions in Ovarian Cancer Screening

In the ovarian cancer screening trials thus far, serum CA-125 has remained the cornerstone of screening; however, this has been found to have low positive predictive value and specificity. Recently, human epididymis protein 4 (HE-4) has been studied as another potential biomarker. CA-125, HE-4, and menopausal status have been combined to create the Risk of Ovarian Malignancy Algorithm (ROMA). The ROMA results are then combined with clinical assessment and results of independent radiological examinations. Much of the research in HE-4 and ROMA has been to evaluate women with pelvic masses to better distinguish between benign and malignant entities.[47] HE-4 was investigated along with CA72-4 and anti-TP53 autoantibodies in the multimodal group of the UKCTOCS trial. The study investigators found that the addition of HE-4, CA72-4, and anti-TP53 autoantibodies did not add value to CA-125 as a first-line test in ovarian cancer screening of asymptomatic postmenopausal women.[48]

There are 2 sources of tumor DNA that can be noninvasively assessed in the circulation: ctDNA and circulating tumor cells (CTCs). CTCs represent intact, often viable, cells that can be purified from blood and distinguished from normal blood cells. Both ctDNA and CTCs have been isolated in blood from women with ovarian cancer, and early studies have shown that there were more CTCs and higher ctDNA levels found in patients with cancer with greater tumor burden.[49–52] CTCs and ctDNA have not yet been evaluated in asymptomatic women without a diagnosis of ovarian cancer.

Serous tubal intraepithelial carcinomas arising in the fallopian tubes have been proposed to be the most likely precursor of ovarian, tubal, and primary peritoneal high-grade serous carcinomas.[53] Obtaining tubal cells via hysteroscopic collection or laparoscopic collection has been shown to be feasible. Further characterization and analysis of these cells are ongoing.[54,55] Ovarian cancers have been found to shed cells in fluids that can be collected cervically via routine Pap tests, and epigenetic and genetic studies can be performed via PCR-based tests.[32,33,56,57]

At this time, there are no effective screening mechanisms in both the low-risk and high-risk population to reduce mortality caused by ovarian cancer. Innovative strategies including various biomarkers, ctDNA, and CTCs, and cells collected via uterine or tubal lavage are being investigated to create an accurate screening test for the asymptomatic general population.

## CERVICAL CANCER

Before the introduction of cervical cancer screening in the mid–twentieth century, cervical cancer was a leading cause of mortality among US women. With the advent of Pap testing, the number of cervical cancer deaths has decreased because of the

**Table 1**
**Summary of recommendations for screening and prevention of gynecologic cancers**

| Cancer Type | Group | Recommendation |
|---|---|---|
| Ovarian cancer | All | Education on signs and symptoms of ovarian cancer<br>Review of family history to identify candidates for genetic testing<br>No screening in asymptomatic low-risk women |
| | BRCA1 carriers | Consider high-risk screening with serial CA-125 and TVUS from age 30 y<br>Risk-reducing salpingo-oophorectomy between 35 and 40 y |
| | BRCA2 carriers | Consider high-risk screening with serial CA-125 and TVUS from age 30 y<br>Risk-reducing salpingo-oophorectomy between 40 and 45 y |
| | BRIP1, RAD51C, RAD51D carriers | Consider high-risk screening with serial CA-125 and TVUS from age 30 y<br>Risk-reducing salpingo-oophorectomy between 40 and 45 y |
| | PALB2 carriers | Consider high-risk screening with serial CA-125 and TVUS from age 30 |
| | Women with Lynch syndrome | Risk-reducing salpingo-oophorectomy with concurrent hysterectomy between 40 and 50 y for MLH1 and MSH2 mutation carriers |
| Endometrial cancer | All | Education on signs and symptoms of endometrial cancer<br>Healthy lifestyle, weight management<br>Management of abnormal uterine bleeding |
| | Women with Lynch syndrome | Consider high-risk screening with endometrial biopsies every 1–2 y from age 30–35 y<br>Consider risk-reducing total hysterectomy at age 40 y or following completion of childbearing |

(continued on next page)

| Table 1 (continued) | | |
|---|---|---|
| Cancer Type | Group | Recommendation |
| Cervical cancer | All | Education on signs and symptoms of cervical cancer |
| | Ages 9–45 y | HPV vaccination |
| | Ages 21–25 y | Cervical cytology screening every 3 y |
| | Ages 25–29 y | Cervical cytology screening every 3 y or HPV-based screening every 5 y |
| | Ages 30–65 y | HPV-based screening or cotesting every 5 y |
| | Ages ≥66 y | HPV-based screening or cotesting if had prior abnormal screening |
| | Immunocompromised women up to age 30y | Cervical cytology screening starting from 1 y after intercourse but no later than age 21 y |
| | Immunocompromised women aged ≥31 y | Cervical cytology and HPV cotesting screening every 5 y |
| Vaginal cancer | All | Education on signs and symptoms of vaginal cancer |
| | Women with history of high-grade cervical dysplasia | Screening for vaginal dysplasia for 25 y after a diagnosis of high-grade cervical dysplasia |
| Vulvar cancer | All | Education on signs and symptoms of vulvar cancer Discussion with patient regarding screening pelvic examinations |

*Abbreviation:* HPV, human papillomavirus.

ability to diagnose preinvasive disease.[58] Despite this, in 2020, there were still an estimated 13,800 new cervical cancer cases and 4290 deaths in the United States.[1]

### Increased Risk of Cervical Cancer: Human Papilloma Virus Infection

Human papillomavirus (HPV) is the known cause of nearly all cases of cervical cancer.[59,60] HPV infections are common within the first decade of sexual activity; however, most of these infections are cleared. Less than 10% of these HPV infections persist, leading to precancerous lesions 5 to 10 years after infection.[59] Expression of the E6 and E7 oncoproteins leads to the degradation of p53 and Rb, thereby allowing HPV to remain in cervical cells, a key step in altering cellular processes and ultimately initiating carcinogenesis.[61] The most common HPV strains that cause cervical cancer are 16, 18, 31, 33, 35, 45, 52, and 58; these strains are responsible for 91% of cervical cancer cases worldwide.[62]

### Prevention of Cervical Cancer in the General Population

In 1942, George Papanicolaou[63] first described the use of cytology as a screening method for cervical cancer. Since then, the incorporation of the Pap test into routine care of women has decreased the burden of cervical cancer across the globe.[58] The latest consensus guidelines have moved to HPV-based testing as the basis for cervical cancer screening.[64] HPV vaccination was first approved in 2006 in the United

States based on data showing its efficacy in preventing HPV persistence and cervical precancer.[65] HPV vaccination is currently recommended for all children and adults aged 9 to 45 years in the United States (see **Table 1**).

### Screening for Low-Risk Individuals

In 2019, the American Society of Colposcopy and Cervical Pathology (ASCCP) published its latest consensus guidelines in conjunction with other national and participating professional organizations. The guiding principles of this fourth version of the ASCCP guidelines include HPV-based screening and management based on risk of cervical intraepithelial neoplasia grade 3 or higher (CIN3+).[64]

For low-risk women, the American Cancer Society (ACS) recommends that primary HPV-based screening be performed every 5 years for women aged 25 to 65 years. A list of the commercially available US Food and Drug Administration (FDA)–approved HPV tests is provided in **Table 2**. When HPV-based screening is not available, then cotesting (HPV testing with cytology) should be performed every 5 years or cytology alone every 3 years.[66–69] Cytology alone is less sensitive than HPV testing and therefore is recommended more frequently.[64] For individuals with HIV or other forms of immunosuppression, initiation and frequency of screening are adjusted given the increased risk (see **Table 1**).

### Management of Abnormal Screening Tests

Based on the risk of CIN3+ associated with their screening results, patients are recommended to undergo either frequent surveillance, colposcopy, or treatment. Data from a population-based study of 1.5 million women undergoing triennial cervical

**Table 2**
**Commercially available US Food and Drug Administration–approved human papilloma virus tests**

| Test | Year Approved | Manufacturer | HPV Genotypes Detected |
|---|---|---|---|
| APTIMA HPV 16 18/45 Genotype Assay | 2011 | Hologic | 16, 18/45 |
| APTIMA HPV Assay | 2011 | Hologic | 16, 18, 31, 33, 35, 39, 45, 51, 52, 56, 58, 59, 66, and 68 |
| BD ONCLARITY HPV ASSAY[a] | 2018 | Becton Dickinson | 16, 18, 31, 33, 35, 39, 45, 51, 52, 56, 58, 59, 66, 68; simultaneous, discrete identification of 16, 18, and 45 |
| Cervista HPV 16/18 | 2009 | Hologic | 16, 18 |
| Cervista HPV HR | 2009 | Hologic | 16, 18, 31, 33, 35, 39, 45, 51, 52, 56, 58, 59, 66, and 68 |
| COBAS HPV Test[a] | 2011 | Roche | 16, 18, 31, 33, 35, 39, 45, 51, 52, 56, 58, 59, 66, and 68 |
| Digene Hybrid Capture 2 | 2001 | Qiagen | 16, 18, 31, 33, 35, 39, 45, 51, 52, 56, 58, 59, 68 |

[a] Approved for primary HPV-based screening.
*Data from* Refs.[64,89,90]

cancer screening at the Kaiser Permanente Northern California from 2003 to 2017 were used to calculate the risk of CIN3+ associated with various test results. These estimates are available for clinicians to access at https://CervixCa.nlm.nih.gov/ RiskTables.[70–72] When the immediate risk of CIN3+ is 4% or greater, immediate treatment or colposcopy is recommended. When the risk is less than 4%, close surveillance is recommended based on the 5-year risk of CIN3+ (**Fig. 3**).[64]

### Future Directions in Cervical Cancer Screening

Screening for cervical cancer involves a pelvic examination with speculum placement and sample collection by a clinician. Given the invasiveness of this process, self-collection has been evaluated. Studies have shown HPV testing from self-collected samples to have similar sensitivity to clinician-collected samples.[73] Urine-based HPV testing has been shown to have good concordance with vaginal and cervical samples in HPV detection.[74–76] These less invasive methods are likely to improve patient compliance and satisfaction, and the authors anticipate that, as these methodologies are validated, these will have the potential to be a part of future cervical cancer screening guidelines.

Given the impact of HPV vaccination in reducing rates of high-grade cervical dysplasia[64] and cancer,[77] we anticipate that vaccination status will affect future screening strategies. As more data are gathered on vaccinated cohorts, women who have completed the HPV vaccination series may be eligible for prolonged screening intervals.[78] As more is learned about CIN3+ risk associated with specific HPV strains, we anticipate that HPV genotyping may be factored into future screening guidelines.[78]

## VAGINAL CANCER

In 2020, there were 6230 new vaginal cancers and 1450 vaginal cancer deaths in the United States.[1] Primary vaginal cancer is a rare disease; most tumors of the vagina are metastatic implants from other primary sites. Most (90%) are squamous cell carcinomas.[79,80]

From the available literature, it seems that the risk of vaginal cancer after hysterectomy is extremely low, and routine screening with vaginal Pap tests should not be

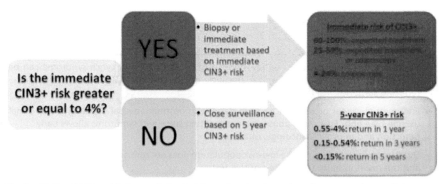

**Fig. 3.** 2019 ASCCP guidelines of CIN3 risk evaluation based on history. When risk is 4% or greater, colposcopy or treatment is recommended. (*Adapted from* Perkins RB, Guido RS, Castle PE, et al. 2019 ASCCP Risk-Based Management Consensus Guidelines for Abnormal Cervical Cancer Screening Tests and Cancer Precursors [published correction appears in J Low Genit Tract Dis. 2020 Oct;24(4):427]. J Low Genit Tract Dis. 2020;24(2):102-131. https://doi.org/10.1097/LGT.0000000000000525; with permission.)

performed for women who do not have a history of high-grade cervical dysplasia or cancer. Women with a history of high-grade cervical dysplasia who have undergone a hysterectomy should continue screening for 25 years following the treatment of high-grade dysplasia.[64] It would be reasonable to expect that future directions for vaginal cancer screening, if any, will be similar to those for cervical cancer screening.

## VULVAR CANCER

Vulvar cancer is the least common gynecologic cancer and accounts for approximately 5% of malignancies of the female genital tract. In 2020, 6120 new vulvar cancers were diagnosed in the United States, with 1350 vulvar cancer deaths.[1] The most common histologic type is squamous cell carcinoma (95%).[81] When identified in early stages, the survival rates are favorable, with 5-year survival of 86% for localized disease.[82] HPV infection of the vulva is associated with usual-type vulvar intraepithelial neoplasia (VIN). When left untreated, approximately 80% of usual-type VIN can progress to vulvar cancer. Differentiated VIN is associated with vulvar dermatologic conditions, such as lichen sclerosus.[83–88] There are no current screening recommendations for vulvar cancer. In the absence of symptoms, a thorough vulvar examination with biopsies as indicated is the only method for early detection of vulvar cancer. Without current screening recommendations and with the low incidence of this disease, it is difficult to anticipate whether this will change in the future.

## SUMMARY

Despite advances in oncologic care, gynecologic cancer continues to be a source of significant morbidity and mortality in women.[1] Cervical cancer is the only gynecologic cancer with an effective screening tool; however, this requires an office visit and is associated with a certain degree of patient discomfort. Abnormal cervical cancer screening can often lead to unnecessary follow-up procedures. There are no current effective screening tests for the other gynecologic malignancies in asymptomatic women. Prevention of risk factors such as obesity and HPV will further reduce the burden of gynecologic cancers. The authors anticipate that the future of gynecologic cancer screening will include a shift toward less invasive, patient-centric, biomarker-driven screening modalities.

## CLINICS CARE POINTS

- Women with cancer genetic predispositions such as *BRCA1/2* and Lynch syndrome can be offered high-risk surveillance for ovarian cancer and/or endometrial cancer as well as risk-reducing surgeries.

- Endometrial cancer presents at an early stage with postmenopausal bleeding or abnormal uterine bleeding. Education about these presenting signs and symptoms allows early detection and improved oncologic outcomes.

- Ovarian cancer screening in the low-risk population does not reduce ovarian cancer mortality and can result in harm from false-positive tests.

- HPV vaccination is effective in preventing HPV infection and persistence, thereby decreasing the development of cervical dysplasia, invasive cervical cancers, and certain types of vulvar and vaginal cancers.

- Accurate identification of high-risk individuals allows the proper implementation of tailored screening mechanisms of various gynecologic malignancies.

## DISCLOSURE

The authors do not have any commercial or financial conflicts of interest.

## REFERENCES

1. Siegel RL, Miller KD, Jemal A. Cancer statistics, 2020. CA Cancer J Clin 2020; 70(1):7–30.
2. Rahib L, Smith BD, Aizenberg R, et al. Projecting Cancer Incidence and Deaths to 2030: The Unexpected Burden of Thyroid, Liver, and Pancreas Cancers in the United States. Cancer Res 2014;74(11):2913–21.
3. Bokhman JV. Two pathogenetic types of endometrial carcinoma. Gynecol Oncol 1983;15(1):10–7.
4. Ueda SM, Kapp DS, Cheung MK, et al. Trends in demographic and clinical characteristics in women diagnosed with corpus cancer and their potential impact on the increasing number of deaths. Am J Obstet Gynecol 2008;198(2):218.e1-6.
5. National Comprehensive Cancer Network. Uterine neoplasms (Version 2.2020). Available at: https://www.nccn.org/professionals/physician_gls/pdf/uterine.pdf. Accessed September 22, 2020.
6. Soliman PT, Bassett RL, Wilson EB, et al. Limited public knowledge of obesity and endometrial cancer risk: what women know. Obstet Gynecol 2008;112(4):835–42.
7. Washington CR, Haggerty A, Ronner W, et al. Knowledge of endometrial cancer risk factors in a general gynecologic population. Gynecol Oncol 2020;158(1): 137–42.
8. Zhang K, Luo Y, Dai H, et al. Effects of Bariatric Surgery on Cancer Risk: Evidence from Meta-analysis. Obes Surg 2020;30(4):1265–72.
9. Jareid M, Thalabard J-C, Aarflot M, et al. Levonorgestrel-releasing intrauterine system use is associated with a decreased risk of ovarian and endometrial cancer, without increased risk of breast cancer. Results from the NOWAC Study. Gynecol Oncol 2018;149(1):127–32.
10. Derbyshire AE, Allen JL, Gittins M, et al. PROgesterone Therapy for Endometrial Cancer prevention in obese women (PROTEC) trial: a feasibility study. Cancer Prev Res 2020. https://doi.org/10.1158/1940-6207.CAPR-20-0248.
11. Allen NE, Key TJ, Dossus L, et al. Endogenous sex hormones and endometrial cancer risk in women in the European Prospective Investigation into Cancer and Nutrition (EPIC). Endocr Relat Cancer 2008;15(2):485–97.
12. Crosbie EJ, Zwahlen M, Kitchener HC, et al. Body mass index, hormone replacement therapy, and endometrial cancer risk: a meta-analysis. Cancer Epidemiol Biomarkers Prev 2010;19(12):3119–30.
13. Arnold M, Pandeya N, Byrnes G, et al. Global burden of cancer attributable to high body-mass index in 2012: a population-based study. Lancet Oncol 2015; 16(1):36–46.
14. Shaw E, Farris M, McNeil J, et al. Obesity and Endometrial Cancer. Recent Results Cancer Res 2016;208:107–36.
15. Barry JA, Azizia MM, Hardiman PJ. Risk of endometrial, ovarian and breast cancer in women with polycystic ovary syndrome: a systematic review and meta-analysis. Hum Reprod Update 2014;20(5):748–58.
16. Fisher B, Costantino JP, Redmond CK, et al. Endometrial cancer in tamoxifen-treated breast cancer patients: findings from the National Surgical Adjuvant Breast and Bowel Project (NSABP) B-14. J Natl Cancer Inst 1994;86(7):527–37.
17. National Comprehensive Cancer Network. Genetic/Familial High-Risk Assessment: Colorectal (Version 1.2021). Available at: https://www.nccn.org/

professionals/physician_gls/pdf/genetics_colon.pdf. Accessed September 22, 2020.

18. Cote ML, Ruterbusch JJ, Olson SH, et al. The Growing Burden of Endometrial Cancer: A Major Racial Disparity Affecting Black Women. Cancer Epidemiol Biomarkers Prev 2015;24(9):1407–15.

19. Doll KM, Khor S, Odem-Davis K, et al. Role of bleeding recognition and evaluation in Black-White disparities in endometrial cancer. Am J Obstet Gynecol 2018; 219(6):593.e1-14.

20. Romano SS, Doll KM. The Impact of Fibroids and Histologic Subtype on the Performance of US Clinical Guidelines for the Diagnosis of Endometrial Cancer among Black Women. Ethn Dis 2020;30(4):543–52.

21. Ries LAG, Young JL, Keel GE, et al (editors). SEER Survival Monograph: Cancer Survival Among Adults: U.S. SEER Program, 1988-2001, Patient and Tumor Characteristics. 2007. Available at: https://seer.cancer.gov/archive/publications/survival/seer_survival_mono_lowres.pdf. Accessed December 24, 2020.

22. Clarke MA, Long BJ, Del Mar Morillo A, et al. Association of Endometrial Cancer Risk With Postmenopausal Bleeding in Women: A Systematic Review and Meta-analysis. JAMA Intern Med 2018;178(9):1210–22.

23. Gerber B, Krause A, Müller H, et al. Ultrasonographic detection of asymptomatic endometrial cancer in postmenopausal patients offers no prognostic advantage over symptomatic disease discovered by uterine bleeding. Eur J Cancer 2001; 37(1):64–71.

24. ACOG Committee Opinion No. 734: The Role of Transvaginal Ultrasonography in Evaluating the Endometrium of Women With Postmenopausal Bleeding. Obstet Gynecol 2018;131(5):e124-e129.

25. Fung MFK, Reid A, Faught W, et al. Prospective longitudinal study of ultrasound screening for endometrial abnormalities in women with breast cancer receiving tamoxifen. Gynecol Oncol 2003;91(1):154–9.

26. Lu KH, Loose DS, Yates MS, et al. Prospective multicenter randomized intermediate biomarker study of oral contraceptive versus depo-provera for prevention of endometrial cancer in women with Lynch syndrome. Cancer Prev Res Phila Pa 2013;6(8):774–81.

27. Jemal A, Ward EM, Johnson CJ, et al. Annual Report to the Nation on the Status of Cancer, 1975-2014, Featuring Survival. J Natl Cancer Inst 2017;109(9). https://doi.org/10.1093/jnci/djx030.

28. Njoku K, Chiasserini D, Jones ER, et al. Urinary Biomarkers and Their Potential for the Non-Invasive Detection of Endometrial Cancer. Front Oncol 2020;10:559016.

29. Bakkum-Gamez JN, Wentzensen N, Maurer MJ, et al. Detection of endometrial cancer via molecular analysis of DNA collected with vaginal tampons. Gynecol Oncol 2015;137(1):14–22.

30. Calis P, Yuce K, Basaran D, et al. Assessment of Cervicovaginal Cancer Antigen 125 Levels: A Preliminary Study for Endometrial Cancer Screening. Gynecol Obstet Invest 2016;81(6):518–22.

31. Heng S, Stephens AN, Jobling TW, et al. Measuring PC activity in endocervical swab may provide a simple and non-invasive method to detect endometrial cancer in post-menopausal women. Oncotarget 2016;7(29):46573–8.

32. Kinde I, Bettegowda C, Wang Y, et al. Evaluation of DNA from the Papanicolaou test to detect ovarian and endometrial cancers. Sci Transl Med 2013;5(167): 167ra4.

33. Wang Y, Li L, Douville C, et al. Evaluation of liquid from the Papanicolaou test and other liquid biopsies for the detection of endometrial and ovarian cancers. Sci Transl Med 2018;10(433). https://doi.org/10.1126/scitranslmed.aap8793.

34. Nair N, Camacho-Vanegas O, Rykunov D, et al. Genomic Analysis of Uterine Lavage Fluid Detects Early Endometrial Cancers and Reveals a Prevalent Landscape of Driver Mutations in Women without Histopathologic Evidence of Cancer: A Prospective Cross-Sectional Study. PLoS Med 2016;13(12):e1002206.

35. Ferlay J, Soerjomataram I, Dikshit R, et al. Cancer incidence and mortality worldwide: sources, methods and major patterns in GLOBOCAN 2012. Int J Cancer 2015;136(5):E359-86.

36. Norquist BM, Harrell MI, Brady MF, et al. Inherited Mutations in Women With Ovarian Carcinoma. JAMA Oncol 2016;2(4):482-90.

37. Pal T, Permuth-Wey J, Betts JA, et al. BRCA1 and BRCA2 mutations account for a large proportion of ovarian carcinoma cases. Cancer 2005;104(12):2807-16.

38. Kuchenbaecker KB, Hopper JL, Barnes DR, et al. Risks of Breast, Ovarian, and Contralateral Breast Cancer for BRCA1 and BRCA2 Mutation Carriers. JAMA 2017;317(23):2402-16.

39. US Preventive Services Task Force, Grossman DC, Curry SJ, et al. Screening for Ovarian Cancer: US Preventive Services Task Force Recommendation Statement. JAMA 2018;319(6):588-94.

40. Buys SS, Partridge E, Black A, et al. Effect of screening on ovarian cancer mortality: the Prostate, Lung, Colorectal and Ovarian (PLCO) Cancer Screening Randomized Controlled Trial. JAMA 2011;305(22):2295-303.

41. Jacobs IJ, Menon U, Ryan A, et al. Ovarian cancer screening and mortality in the UK Collaborative Trial of Ovarian Cancer Screening (UKCTOCS): a randomised controlled trial. Lancet 2016;387(10022):945-56.

42. National Comprehensive Cancer Network. Genetic/Familial High-Risk Assessment: Breast, Ovarian, and Pancreatic (Version 1.2021). Available at: https://www.nccn.org/professionals/physician_gls/pdf/genetics_bop.pdf. Accessed September 22, 2020.

43. Kauff ND, Domchek SM, Friebel TM, et al. Risk-Reducing Salpingo-Oophorectomy for the Prevention of BRCA1- and BRCA2-Associated Breast and Gynecologic Cancer: A Multicenter, Prospective Study. J Clin Oncol 2008; 26(8):1331-7.

44. Finch APM, Lubinski J, Møller P, et al. Impact of oophorectomy on cancer incidence and mortality in women with a BRCA1 or BRCA2 mutation. J Clin Oncol 2014;32(15):1547-53.

45. Rosenthal AN, Fraser LSM, Philpott S, et al. Evidence of Stage Shift in Women Diagnosed With Ovarian Cancer During Phase II of the United Kingdom Familial Ovarian Cancer Screening Study. J Clin Oncol 2017;35(13):1411-20.

46. Skates SJ, Greene MH, Buys SS, et al. Early Detection of Ovarian Cancer using the Risk of Ovarian Cancer Algorithm with Frequent CA125 Testing in Women at Increased Familial Risk - Combined Results from Two Screening Trials. Clin Cancer Res 2017;23(14):3628-37.

47. Moore RG, Miller MC, Disilvestro P, et al. Evaluation of the diagnostic accuracy of the risk of ovarian malignancy algorithm in women with a pelvic mass. Obstet Gynecol 2011;118(2 Pt 1):280-8.

48. Gentry-Maharaj A, Blyuss O, Ryan A, et al. Multi-Marker Longitudinal Algorithms Incorporating HE4 and CA125 in Ovarian Cancer Screening of Postmenopausal Women. Cancers 2020;12(7). https://doi.org/10.3390/cancers12071931.

49. Pearl ML, Zhao Q, Yang J, et al. Prognostic analysis of invasive circulating tumor cells (iCTCs) in epithelial ovarian cancer. Gynecol Oncol 2014;134(3):581–90.
50. Zhang X, Li H, Yu X, et al. Analysis of circulating tumor cells in ovarian cancer and their clinical value as a biomarker. Cell Physiol Biochem 2018;48(5):1983–94.
51. Vanderstichele A, Busschaert P, Smeets D, et al. Chromosomal Instability in Cell-Free DNA as a Highly Specific Biomarker for Detection of Ovarian Cancer in Women with Adnexal Masses. Clin Cancer Res 2017;23(9):2223–31.
52. Pereira E, Camacho-Vanegas O, Anand S, et al. Personalized Circulating Tumor DNA Biomarkers Dynamically Predict Treatment Response and Survival In Gynecologic Cancers. PLoS One 2015;10(12):e0145754.
53. Kurman RJ, Shih I-M. Molecular pathogenesis and extraovarian origin of epithelial ovarian cancer–shifting the paradigm. Hum Pathol 2011;42(7):918–31.
54. Pramanik S, Yang E, Wu W. Cytologic studies of in vivo fallopian tube specimens in patients undergoing salpingo-oophorectomy. CytoJournal 2020;17:19.
55. Chen H, Klein R, Arnold S, et al. Tubal Cytology of the Fallopian Tube as a Promising Tool for Ovarian Cancer Early Detection. J Vis Exp Jove 2017;125. https://doi.org/10.3791/55887.
56. Ersoy E, Kashikar RM. Psammoma bodies in Papanicolaou tests and associated factors to predict an underlying malignancy: a clinicopathological analysis of 10 cases. J Am Soc Cytopathol 2020;9(4):266–71.
57. Wu T-I, Huang R-L, Su P-H, et al. Ovarian cancer detection by DNA methylation in cervical scrapings. Clin Epigenetics 2019;11(1):166.
58. Saslow D, Solomon D, Lawson HW, et al. American Cancer Society, American Society for Colposcopy and Cervical Pathology, and American Society for Clinical Pathology Screening Guidelines for the Prevention and Early Detection of Cervical Cancer. Am J Clin Pathol 2012;137(4):516–42.
59. Schiffman M, Castle PE, Jeronimo J, et al. Human papillomavirus and cervical cancer. Lancet 2007;370(9590):890–907.
60. Muñoz N. Human papillomavirus and cancer: the epidemiological evidence. J Clin Virol 2000;19(1–2):1–5.
61. Szymonowicz KA, Chen J. Biological and clinical aspects of HPV-related cancers. Cancer Biol Med 2020;17(4):864–78.
62. de Sanjose S, Quint WG, Alemany L, et al. Human papillomavirus genotype attribution in invasive cervical cancer: a retrospective cross-sectional worldwide study. Lancet Oncol 2010;11(11):1048–56.
63. Papanicolaou GN. A NEW PROCEDURE FOR STAINING VAGINAL SMEARS. Science 1942;95(2469):438–9.
64. Perkins RB, Guido RS, Castle PE, et al. 2019 ASCCP Risk-Based Management Consensus Guidelines for Abnormal Cervical Cancer Screening Tests and Cancer Precursors. J Low Genit Tract Dis 2020;24(2):102–31. https://doi.org/10.1097/LGT.0000000000000525.
65. Gattoc L, Nair N, Ault K. Human Papillomavirus Vaccination. Obstet Gynecol Clin North Am 2013;40(2):177–97.
66. Fontham ETH, Wolf AMD, Church TR, et al. Cervical cancer screening for individuals at average risk: 2020 guideline update from the American Cancer Society. CA Cancer J Clin 2020;70(5):321–46.
67. Liu G, Sharma M, Tan N, et al. HIV-positive women have higher risk of human papilloma virus infection, precancerous lesions, and cervical cancer. AIDS 2018;32(6):795–808.
68. Panel on Opportunistic Infections in Adults and Adolescents with HIV. Guidelines for the prevention and treatment of opportunistic infections in adults and

adolescents with HIV: recommendations from the Centers for Disease Control and Prevention, the National Institutes of Health, and the HIV Medicine Association of the Infectious Diseases Society of America. Available at: http://aidsinfo.nih. gov/contentfiles/lvguidelines/adult_oi.pdf. Accessed December 20, 2020.

69. Moscicki A-B, Flowers L, Huchko MJ, et al. Guidelines for Cervical Cancer Screening in Immunosuppressed Women Without HIV Infection. J Low Genit Tract Dis 2019;23(2):87–101.

70. Cheung LC, Egemen D, Chen X, et al. 2019 ASCCP Risk-Based Management Consensus Guidelines: Methods for Risk Estimation, Recommended Management, and Validation. J Low Genit Tract Dis 2020;24(2):90–101.

71. Egemen D, Cheung LC, Chen X, et al. Risk Estimates Supporting the 2019 ASCCP Risk-Based Management Consensus Guidelines. J Low Genit Tract Dis 2020;24(2):132–43.

72. Demarco M, Egemen D, Raine-Bennett TR, et al. A Study of Partial Human Papillomavirus Genotyping in Support of the 2019 ASCCP Risk-Based Management Consensus Guidelines. J Low Genit Tract Dis 2020;24(2):144–7.

73. Snijders PJF, Verhoef VMJ, Arbyn M, et al. High-risk HPV testing on self-sampled versus clinician-collected specimens: a review on the clinical accuracy and impact on population attendance in cervical cancer screening. Int J Cancer 2013;132(10):2223–36.

74. Tranberg M, Jensen JS, Bech BH, et al. Urine collection in cervical cancer screening - analytical comparison of two HPV DNA assays. BMC Infect Dis 2020;20(1):926.

75. Cho H-W, Ouh Y-T, Hong JH, et al. Comparison of urine, self-collected vaginal swab, and cervical swab samples for detecting human papillomavirus (HPV) with Roche Cobas HPV, Anyplex II HPV, and RealTime HR-S HPV assay. J Virol Methods 2019;269:77–82.

76. Lichter K, Krause D, Xu J, et al. Adjuvant HPV vaccination with surgical excision to prevent recurrent CIN2+: A systematic review and meta-analysis. Featured Poster Session presented at the: Society of Gynecologic Oncology Annual Meeting; March 2020.

77. Lei J, Ploner A, Elfström KM, et al. HPV Vaccination and the Risk of Invasive Cervical Cancer. N Engl J Med 2020;383(14):1340-1348.

78. Liverani CA, Di Giuseppe J, Giannella L, et al. Cervical Cancer Screening Guidelines in the Postvaccination Era: Review of the Literature. J Oncol 2020;2020: 8887672.

79. Hacker NF, Eifel PJ, van der Velden J. Cancer of the vagina. Int J Gynaecol Obstet 2015;131(Suppl 2):S84–7.

80. Khadraoui H, Thappa S, Smith M, et al. Age-associated trends of vulvar cancer in the US. Menopause N Y N 2020. https://doi.org/10.1097/GME. 0000000000001687.

81. Alkatout I, Schubert M, Garbrecht N, et al. Vulvar cancer: epidemiology, clinical presentation, and management options. Int J Womens Health 2015;7:305–13.

82. American Cancer Society. Cancer Facts & Figures 2020. Atlanta Am Cancer Soc; 2020.

83. Committee on Gynecologic Practice of American College Obstetricians and Gynecologists. ACOG Committee Opinion No. 509: Management of vulvar intraepithelial neoplasia. Obstet Gynecol 2011;118(5):1192–4.

84. US Preventive Services Task Force, Bibbins-Domingo K, Grossman DC, et al. Screening for Gynecologic Conditions With Pelvic Examination: US Preventive Services Task Force Recommendation Statement. JAMA 2017;317(9):947.

85. Qaseem A, Humphrey LL, Harris R, et al. Clinical Guidelines Committee of the American College of Physicians. Screening pelvic examination in adult women: a clinical practice guideline from the American College of Physicians. Ann Intern Med 2014;161(1):67–72.

86. American Academy of Family Physicians. Summary of Recommendations for Clinical Preventive Services. Available at: https://www.aafp.org/dam/AAFP/documents/patient_care/clinical_recommendations/cps-recommendations.pdf. Accessed December 24, 2020.

87. Conry JA, Brown H. Well-Woman Task Force: Components of the Well-Woman Visit. Obstet Gynecol 2015;126(4):697–701.

88. ACOG Committee Opinion No. 755 Summary: Well-Woman Visit. Obstet Gynecol 2018;132(4):1084–5.

89. U.S. Food & Drug Administration. Nucleic Acid Based Tests. Available at: https://www.fda.gov/medical-devices/vitro-diagnostics/nucleic-acid-based-tests. Accessed December 29, 2020.

90. Salazar KL, Duhon DJ, Olsen R, et al. A review of the FDA-approved molecular testing platforms for human papillomavirus. J Am Soc Cytopathol 2019;8(5):284–92.

# Contraceptive Technology
## Present and Future

Allison L. Gilbert, MD, MPH[a], Barbara L. Hoffman, MD[b],*

## KEYWORDS

• Novel • Patch • Ring • Progestin-only • Spermicide • Intrauterine • Emergency

## KEY POINTS

• New choices that include a vaginal ring, transdermal patch, progestin-only pill, and spermicide expand options for those desiring contraception. Additional technologies lay on the horizon.

## INTRODUCTION

From 2015 to 2017 in the United States, nearly two-thirds of sexually active individuals capable of becoming pregnant were actively using a contraceptive method, and nearly all have used at least 1 contraceptive method in their lifetime.[1,2] To expand options for those desiring birth control, new methods include a vaginal ring, transdermal patch, progestin-only pill, and spermicide. Additionally, updated insertion methods for current intrauterine contraceptives (IUCs), depot medroxyprogesterone acetate, and the progestin-only implant aim to enhance access and safety.

Although existing methods are safer and offer more choice than ever before, exciting new contraceptive technologies lay on the horizon. Also, using existing contraceptives in innovative ways aims to decrease barriers to care. Some of the novel technologies include new oral estrogens, contraceptive vaginal rings (CVRs), IUCs, contraceptive delivery methods, multipurpose prevention technologies, and nonsteroidal monoclonal antibodies.

A. L. Gilbert, has no conflicts of interest or financial ties to disclose.
B. L. Hoffman, has no relationships with the medical industry to disclose.
Funding source includes McGraw-Hill Education.
[a] Southwestern Women's Surgical Center, 8616 Greenville Avenue, #101, Dallas, TX 75243, USA;
[b] Department of Obstetrics and Gynecology, University of Texas Southwestern Medical Center, Rm H6.204, Mail Code 9032, 5323 Harry Hines Boulevard, Dallas, TX 75390, USA
* Corresponding author.
E-mail address: Barbara.hoffman@utsouthwestern.edu

Obstet Gynecol Clin N Am 48 (2021) 723–735
https://doi.org/10.1016/j.ogc.2021.07.001
0889-8545/21/© 2021 Elsevier Inc. All rights reserved.

obgyn.theclinics.com

## SOME AVAILABLE METHODS
### Contraceptive Vaginal Rings

NuvaRing is a flexible, clear CVR that measures 54 mm in diameter and 4 mm in cross-section. Its core releases ethinyl estradiol (EE) and the progestin etonogestrel. Annovera is a new CVR that releases EE and the progestin segesterone acetate. Colored white, it measures 56 mm in diameter and 8.4 mm in cross-section.

For both devices, hormones are slowly released and then absorbed across the vaginal epithelium. Either ring is initially inserted within 5 days of menses onset. After 3 weeks of use, it is removed for 1 week to allow withdrawal bleeding. The Nuvaring is single use, and after that 1 week, a new ring is placed. In contrast, after removal and washing, the same Annovera ring is reinserted after 1 week for another 3 weeks of use. One ring can function for 13 such cycles.[3] Continuous use is an option with the NuvaRing, and a new ring is inserted immediately after removal of the old ring at 3-week intervals. More studies are needed to determine the safety and efficacy of continuous Annovera.

With insertion, the ring is compressed and advanced into the vagina, but no specific final orientation within the vagina is required. Patient satisfaction is high with this method, although vaginitis, ring-related events, and leukorrhea are more common than with combination oral contraceptives (COCs).[4,5] A ring may be used concurrently with vaginal medications or with a tampon. However, with Annovera, the concurrent use of a miconazole suppository increases systemic hormone concentrations. These levels are not altered by miconazole cream, and thus cream antifungals or oral fluconazole are preferred treatment for candidiasis.[6] Partners may feel the ring during intercourse. If bothersome, the ring may be removed for intercourse, but should be replaced within 3 hours for the Nuvaring and within 2 hours for Annovera to maintain efficacy. Annovera has not been studied for use in those with body mass index of more than 29 kg/m$^2$.

### Transdermal Patches

The Ortho Evra patch and its generic Xulane each contain EE and the progestin norelgestromin. A newer patch, Twirla, releases EE and levonorgestrel (LNG). Either patch type may be applied to the buttocks, upper outer arm, lower abdomen, or upper torso, but the breasts are avoided. Rates of application site skin reaction are low.[7,8] If a patch is so poorly adhered that it requires reinforcement with tape, it should be replaced. Women can wear the patch in saunas and whirlpools without decreased efficacy.[9,10] However, with Twirla, swimming is limited to 30 minutes.

The initiation of the patch is the same as for COCs, and a new patch is applied weekly for 3 weeks, followed by 1 patch-free week to allow withdrawal bleeding. In general, the transdermal patches and vaginal rings produce metabolic changes, side effects, and efficacy rates comparable with those with COC pills. However, the Ortho Evra patch has been associated with a higher venous thromboembolism (VTE) risk in some but not all studies.[11] Labeling for the patch states that the risk for VTE may be higher compared with COCs, and relative risk estimates range from 1.2 to 2.2. In addition, obesity—90 kg or greater—may be associated with a higher risk for patch contraceptive failure.[12]

From early data, Twirla may avoid these concerns. In a randomized trial, the VTE rates between Twirla and COCs were comparable.[7] Additionally, contraceptive efficacy was similar between obese and normal-weight users.

### Progestin-Only Pills

Also called mini-pills, this group contains norethindrone-only, drospirenone-only, and desogestrel-only pills. Traditional progestin-only pills contain norethindrone. Each pill provides 0.35 mg of hormone and is taken daily and continuously, with no dosing breaks. This specific drug does not reliably inhibit ovulation, and efficacy stems from cervical mucus thickening and endometrial atrophy. Because mucus changes are not sustained, these pills are best taken at the same time each day. If the pill is taken even 3 hours late, which is called the missed pill window, a second form of contraception is used for the next 48 hours. These hindrances have limited progestin-only pill popularity and increased typical use pregnancy rates compared with COCs.

A new drospirenone-only pill is marketed as Slynd and delivers 4 mg of hormone. It is taken for 24 consecutive days in a 28-day cycle. Progestin withdrawal during the last 4 days aims to minimize midcycle bleeding.[13] Both drospirenone and desogestrel pills reliably inhibit ovulation in addition to the traditional mucus and endometrium changes. Advantageously, Slynd offers a longer, 24-hour missed-pill window, which mirrors that of COC pills.[14]

Drospirenone is structurally similar to spironolactone. It displays antiandrogenic activity, provides an antialdosterone action to minimize water retention, and has antimineralocorticoid properties that may, in theory, cause potassium retention and hyperkalemia.[15] Thus, contraindications are renal or adrenal insufficiency in addition to traditional progestin contraindications. Serum potassium level monitoring is recommended in the first month for patients chronically treated with any drug associated with potassium retention. These include nonsteroidal anti-inflammatory drugs, angiotensin-converting enzyme inhibitors, angiotensin II antagonists, heparin, aldosterone antagonists, and potassium-sparing diuretics.

Last in this group is a desogestrel-only pill that contains 0.075 mg of hormone and is used daily and continuously. Its missed pill window is 12 hours. This type of contraception is not available in the United States.

### Subcutaneous Depot Medroxyprogesterone

A subcutaneous version of depot medroxyprogesterone acetate that supplies 104 mg, Depo-SubQ Provera 104, was approved by the US Food and Drug Administration (FDA) in 2004. It has been widely unavailable owing to inconsistent stocking and prohibitive costs. Despite these factors, data consistently show this form to be safe, effective, and acceptable to both users and health care providers. A renewed interest in this self-administered method has emerged to help expand options, decrease barriers to access, and increase reproductive autonomy through self-managed care.[16]

### Spermicides

Traditional spermicides contain nonoxynol-9 and are sold over the counter in various forms. They provide a chemical spermicidal action and a physical barrier to sperm penetration. Their duration of maximal effectiveness is usually no more than 1 hour, and these modalities do not offer protection against sexually transmitted infection.

In 2020, a vaginal contraceptive gel containing lactic acid, citric acid, and potassium bitartrate was approved by the FDA as Phexxi. As an acidifying agent, it resists the buffering effect of semen, which is alkaline. This factor allows the vagina's normally acidic pH to work as a natural spermicide.[17] In a phase III trial, its typical use efficacy was 86%.[18] This vaginal pH modulator can be used with latex or polyurethane condoms and with diaphragms. It is also compatible with antifungal agents for vaginal candidiasis. Of caveats, common adverse reactions with Phexxi were vulvovaginal burning or pruritus, mycotic infection, urinary tract infection, and bacterial vaginosis.[18]

Ideally, either spermicidal agent is deposited high in the vagina up to 1 hour before coitus. Thereafter, each must be reinserted before repeat intercourse.

## Progestin Implants

Implants are among the most effective contraceptive methods. These thin, pliable, progestin-containing cylinders are placed subdermally on the inner upper arm to release contraceptive hormone over several years. Implants vary in their insertion technique, and the manufacturer's instructions should be consulted. After their expiration date, implants are removed and may be replaced at the same site or in the opposite arm.

Nexplanon is a single-rod etonogestrel implant that releases at least 30 μg of hormone daily and may be used for 3 years. Its inserter's design aids correct subdermal positioning and averting deeper placement. Nexplanon replaced Implanon, which is still approved by the FDA but no longer distributed by the manufacturer.

LNG implants are 2-rod systems available outside the United States and contain a total progestin dose of 150 mg. Jadelle provides contraception for 5 years. It is approved by the FDA but not marketed in the United States. A second device is the Sino-implant II, which provides 3 years of contraception.[19]

In addition to potential hormonal side effects, the implants themselves can cause adverse events. First, nonpalpable devices are not uncommon and require imaging for localization before attempted removal. Nexplanon is radiopaque and can be imaged by 2-dimensional x-ray views. Implanon is not radiopaque, and sonography using a 10- to 15-MHz linear array transducer or MR imaging is needed. Rarely, an implant can migrate to distant sites such as the lung. If imaging fails to locate an implant, etonogestrel blood levels can help to verify that the implant is indeed in situ. This assay must be coordinated with the manufacturer (1–877–888–4231).

Second, serious neurovascular injury can infrequently complicate implant insertions and removals.[20,21] An implant inserted too deeply or removals that involve wide or deep exploration are mechanisms of injury. Thus, implants positioned deep in the muscle or near neurovascular structures are best removed by surgeons with an understanding of upper arm anatomy.

As 1 response, a new manufacturer's insertion method has moved the placement site away from the biceps groove, which lies between the biceps and triceps muscle. Near this groove, the medial antebrachial cutaneous nerve, medial brachial cutaneous nerve, ulnar nerve, and basilica vein typically run. To avoid these structures, the new site is positioned away from the groove to a more medial site that lies closer to the posterior arm. Specifically, the insertion site is marked 8 to 10 cm proximal to the humerus' medial condyle and 3 to 5 cm posterior to the groove between biceps and triceps muscles.[22] A second mark is placed 4 cm proximal to the first and serves as a guide for the insertion path along the arm's long axis.

## Intrauterine Contraceptives

Five IUCs are currently approved for use in the United States. These continually elute either copper or LNG. All have a flexible, T-shaped polyethylene frame that is compounded with barium to render them radiopaque. The LNG-releasing intrauterine systems (LNG-IUSs) are similarly shaped, but each differs by size, string color, longevity, and the presence or absence of a silver band at the junction of the stem and arms (**Table 1**). Among these, smaller-sized devices were designed to better fit a nulliparous uterus; however, full-sized IUCs are still suitable for nulliparas. The silver band is echogenic and allows the similarly shaped LNG-IUSs to be differentiated sonographically. In contrast, the copper device, the CuT380A IUC named ParaGard, contains a thin copper strand wound around its stem and a copper bracelet on each arm.

IUC insertion traditionally has followed a menstrual cycle or complete uterine involution after a pregnancy has ended. This is termed interval placement. Instead,

**Table 1**
**Properties of some intrauterine devices**

| Active Agent | Quantity of Active Agent | Width × Height (mm) | Inserter Tube Diameter (mm) | Duration of Use (y) | String Color | Silver Ring | Brand Name |
|---|---|---|---|---|---|---|---|
| LNG | 52 mg | 32 × 32 | 4.4 | 5 | Tan | No | Mirena |
| LNG | 52 mg | 32 × 32 | 4.8 | 6 | Blue | No | Liletta |
| LNG | 19.5 mg | 28 × 30 | 3.8 | 5 | Blue | Yes | Kyleena |
| LNG | 13.5 mg | 28 × 30 | 3.8 | 3 | Tan | Yes | Skyla, Jaydess |
| LNG | 14 µg / 20 µg | 1.2 × 30 / 1.6 × 35 (frameless) | 3.0 | 3 / 5 | Blue | No | Fibroplant[a] |
| Copper | 380 mm² | 32 × 36 | 4.4 | 10 | White | No | ParaGard |
| Copper | 380 mm² | 30 × 24 | 3.7 | 5 | Blue | No | Mona Lisa Mini[a] |
| Copper | 175 mm² | 30 × 32 | 3.7 | 5 | Blue | No | VeraCept[a] |
| Copper | 300 mm² | 12-, 15-, or 18-mm diameters | 3.2 | 5 | Blue | No | Ballerine[a] |

*Abbreviation:* LNG, levonorgestrel.
[a] Not currently available in the United States.

immediate placement can follow reasonable exclusion of pregnancy, early pregnancy loss, aspiration abortion, or delivery in the absence of overt infection or hemorrhage.[23,24] Early insertion 1 week after mifepristone and completed medication abortion has been described.[25,26] These options aim to expand contraceptive access for those desiring long-acting reversible contraception. Compared with interval insertion, the IUC expulsion rate is higher with immediate placement, defined as the first 10 minutes after placenta delivery. However, the number of women in immediate placement groups who ultimately receive and retain an IUC is greater than in groups scheduled for interval placement, because some women fail to return for insertion.[27,28]

## FUTURE CONTRACEPTION

Future contraceptive technologies seek to provide options that are highly effective, widely available, easy to use, cost efficient, and well-tolerated compared with currently available methods. In their development, patient choice and reproductive autonomy are ideally emphasized. This discussion explores potentially new contraceptive technologies and innovative ways in which existing methods may be used to lower barriers to care and promote a more user-controlled experience.

### Novel Technologies

### Oral estrogens

COCs contain an estrogen and progestin to improve contraceptive efficacy and bleeding profiles compared with progestin-only pills. EE has been the main estrogen used in the United States since the 1960s. In contrast, many different progestins are available. Although lower doses (10 mg, 20 mg, or 30 mg) are now more commonly selected, EE is still associated with an increased risk of VTE and cardiovascular disease. Other orally available estrogens such as estradiol (E2) and estetrol have high patient satisfaction scores yet decrease the coagulation markers and hemostatic effects commonly seen with EE.

Estelle is an oral COC containing 15 mg estetrol and 3 mg drospirenone. Estetrol is a naturally occurring estrogen that is produced by human fetal liver cells during pregnancy. Its half-life is 20 to 28 hours.[29] Phase II studies of estetrol show a favorable VTE risk profile compared with EE. Estelle completed its phase III trial in the United States and Canada in 2018 and was submitted to the FDA for review in July 2020 (ClinicalTrials.gov identifier NCT02817841). Its Pearl Index (defined as the number of contraceptive failures per 100 person-years of exposure) is 2.41, which is comparable with the most recent FDA-approved contraceptives. If approved, Estelle could provide a safer estrogen-containing contraceptive for daily pill users.[30,31]

### Contraceptive vaginal rings

Both of the CVRs described elsewhere in this article (NuvaRing and Annovera) contain EE to aid ovulation inhibition and limit breakthrough bleeding. Compared with these rings, one using E2 may offer significant advantages by decreasing coagulation markers and hemostatic effects when administered transdermally or tranvaginally.[32] For example, promising dose-finding studies have examined E2 in combination with segesterone acetate (Nestorone).[33,34] This progestin has low oral bioavailability but potent activity when applied vaginally, transdermally, or subdermally.[35] Segesterone acetate-only containing rings have been studied, but had follicular development and unfavorable breakthrough bleeding. These limitations led to the addition of E2.[36] A 90-day CVR releasing E2 200 μg/d and segesterone acetate 200 μg/d is undergoing a phase IIb trial to determine contraceptive efficacy (ClinicalTrials.gov identifier NCT03432416).

No progestin-only vaginal rings are currently available in the United States. Progering, a progesterone-only vaginal ring, is available in some Latin American and African countries and is being studied in India, but only as an adjunct to the lactational amenorrhea method.[37]

A new, 28-day, trimegestone-containing progestin-only vaginal ring that offers high efficacy and an improved bleeding profile is under development.[38] Trimegestone is a potent progestin that acts on the endometrium. It has no estrogenic, androgenic, or glucocorticoid effects, and modest antiandrogenic and antimineralocorticoid effects. A recent dose-finding trial showed promising results for ovulation inhibition that was comparable with the newer drosperinone- and desogestrel-only pills, described earlier. Rates of breakthrough bleeding were not examined in this study. Further studies showing contraceptive effect and tolerability are still needed.

Modulation of the progestin receptor is another potential avenue for estrogen-free contraceptives. A ulipristal acetate (UPA)-containing CVR used continuously for 3 months is under development by the Population Council. UPA is a progesterone-receptor modulator that seems to have contraceptive activity by ovulation inhibition.[39] UPA is currently FDA approved as an oral emergency contraceptive and successfully postpones the luteinizing hormone surge and subsequent follicle rupture when taken within 5 days of unprotected intercourse.

Although promising, endometrial glandular changes were noted with chronic UPA use and termed progesterone-receptor modulator–associated endometrial changes. Although UPA used for emergency contraception has not been implicated, chronic oral UPA use for leiomyoma management has been also associated with rare liver failure.[40] Further studies are needed to determine its long-term safety.

A novel nonhormonal CVR is in development. Ovaprene (ferrous gluconate/ascorbic acid) is a monthly nonhormonal vaginal ring (ClinicalTrials.gov identifier NCT03598088). The ring has a knitted polymer barrier at its center to impair sperm motility and to physically block sperm entry into the cervical canal.[29]

### Intrauterine contraceptives

At least 2 new nonhormonal, copper-containing, IUCs are currently being studied in the United States. The first is marketed as the Mona Lisa NT Cu380 Mini. This T-shaped device contains 380 mm$^2$ of copper wire wrapped around its stem and measures 30 mm × 24 mm. This smaller frame may be more desirable for nulliparas than the 36 mm × 32 mm dimensions of ParaGard (see **Table 1**). The Mona Lisa NT Cu380 Mini offers 5 years of efficacy. It is approved for use in Europe, and a large multicenter randomized trial in the United States is underway (CinicalTrials.gov identifier NCT03124160). Completion is expected in late 2021.

A lower-dose, T-shaped, copper-containing IUC is marketed as VeraCept (VC175). This device presents a 175-mm$^2$ copper surface via small beads attached to a flexible nitinol frame that measures 30 mm × 32 mm. Nitinol is a shape memory, nickel–titanium alloy wire. Compared with the CuT380A, the novel frame of VC175 may result in less insertional pain, fewer expulsions, and a lower discontinuation rate from heavy bleeding and cramping.[41] Data from a recent phase II study shows efficacy and safety (ClinicalTrials.gov identifier NCT02446821).[42] A phase III clinical trial is currently ongoing (ClinicalTrials.gov identifier NCT03633799).

Many different IUCs are currently available outside of the United States. Their innovative designs may one day be available here. One such device is a copper IUC that also contains indomethacin. The latter aims to decrease menstrual-related complaints commonly associated with Paragard.[43,44]

Another design is the copper intrauterine ball marketed as Ballerine. The intrauterine ball has a nitinol frame with 17 copper spheres attached and is available in 3 sizes with a 12-, 15-, or 18-mm diameter. Its flexible spherical shape may cause less cramping and lower the perforation risk.[43] Contraceptive efficacy lasts 5 years.

Frameless IUCs have been under development since the 1980s and capitalize on the concept that uterine cavities differ in shape and size among women and during a menstrual cycle. Frameless IUCs allow the greatest flexibility. Both hormonal and nonhormonal versions of the frameless IUC currently exist but are not approved for use in the United States. One device, marketed as GyneFix, contains copper beads attached to a polypropylene thread that is, anchored into the myometrium with the inserter. Another device, marketed as Fibroplant, contains LNG and is similar in shape and size to Nexplanon. It is attached to a permanent suture, which is knotted on one end and implanted into the myometrium.[43]

### Delivery systems

Hormonal contraceptives generally provide suitable efficacy. However, these require either frequent dosing, which can lead to poor compliance, or delivery by a health care provider, which can be a barrier to care. User-controlled delivery systems aim to bypass these limitations. Some currently in development include a new transdermal patch, a longer lasting oral contraceptive, and contraceptive jewelry.

The currently available transdermal patch is replaced once weekly and can be seen when applied. Instead, a biodegradable, microneedle-containing patch that can be painlessly applied to the skin is under development. Once the applied patch is removed, the dermally placed microneedles separate from the patch to biodegrade and slowly release their hormone over time. This provides a longer acting and more discrete method. One investigational patch couples LNG and the biodegradable polymers polyactic acid and polylactic-co-glycolic acid.[45]

A once-monthly oral contraceptive pill could improve compliance for those who prefer oral contraceptives. Unfortunately, most oral medications are eliminated quickly owing to short gastrointestinal transit times. One answer may be a gelatin capsule that, once ingested, expands and stays in the stomach for up to 3 weeks. This delivery system has been proven in 1- and 2-week intervals for infectious disease medications.[46]

Pharmaceutical jewelry may increase acceptability and adherence to use. Transdermal patches containing LNG have been incorporated into an earring, ring, necklace, and wristwatch. Thus far, this jewelry has only been tested in animal models. When applied daily—16 hours on and 8 hours off to simulate taking jewelry off at night—serum LNG concentrations remained above the human contraceptive threshold.[47] This method may be a fun solution to improving the acceptability of transdermal drug delivery and to increasing compliance.

### Multipurpose prevention technologies

These products address multiple sexual and reproductive health needs, such as contraception and sexually transmitted infection prevention. Long-acting or on-demand multipurpose prevention technologies are under development. Long-acting multipurpose prevention technologies include vaginal rings, injectables, and oral pills.[48] On-demand multipurpose prevention technologies include topical gels to be used alone or in concert with barrier methods.[49]

Two investigational long-acting vaginal rings are embedded with an antiretroviral medication to prevent HIV-1 transmission and with LNG to prevent unintended pregnancy. Rings containing dapivirine plus LNG or tenofovir plus LNG are effective during

60- and 90-day periods, respectively.[49,50] Another long-acting formulation under study couples the pre-exposure prophylaxis medication rilpivirine with an injectable contraceptive such as depot medroxyprogesterone acetate. One investigational on-demand multipurpose prevention technologies is a tenofovir gel that helps prevent HIV-1 and herpes simplex virus-2 transmission. This gel could be used in combination with a spermicide or as an adjunct to barrier contraception.[49]

### Nonsteroidal technologies
Nonsteroidal contraceptives that use antisperm monoclonal antibodies are being developed. One such technology uses a film that dissolves on contact with vaginal mucosa to deliver on-demand contraception.[51] This technology could be used alone or in combination with other monoclonal antibodies directed against sexually transmitted infections. Vaginal rings may be another delivery system for monoclonal antibody technology.[52]

## Novel Uses of Existing Contraceptives

### Intrauterine emergency contraception
The copper-containing ParaGard is the only IUC used for emergency contraception in the United States. New evidence suggests that the 52-mg LNG-IUS may be a noninferior option when placed within 5 days of unprotected intercourse. In a randomized trial, more than 600 women were assigned to receive one of these for emergency contraception. Pregnancy occurred in 1 participant in the LNG-IUS group and in none of the CuT380A group (0.3% v. 0.0%).[53] As a greater number IUC users select the LNG-IUS than the copper IUC in the United States, the addition of the LNG-IUS to the list of emergency contraception options may allow users that long-acting reversible contraception form. Additionally, LNG-IUS use for emergency contraception could decrease barriers for immediate IUC placement for patients who desire the device, but in whom pregnancy cannot be reasonably excluded owing recent unprotected intercourse.

Typically placed within 5 days of unprotected intercourse, the CuT380A IUD may be effective for up to 14 days for emergency contraception. In a recent study of 134 women with the CuT380A IUC placed 6 to 14 days after unprotected intercourse, no pregnancies occurred within 4 weeks of IUC placement.[54]

### IUC self-removal
IUCs are effective, safe, and popular, but require a health care provider visit for placement and removal. This limitation is one reason that some people do not consider this method.[55] Patient-reported barriers to removal include removal costs, inaccessibility to appointments, and provider resistance to removal.[56]

In response, an emerging practice is IUC self-removal. It is unknown how many people choose this option. One study showed a success rate of 20% for those who tried. Success was associated with the length of the strings, and each additional centimeter of length increased success by more than 50%. More than one-half of participants were more likely to recommend IUC use to a friend once they knew it was possible to remove their own device.[57] However, another study showed no difference in IUC uptake, satisfaction, or discontinuation rates for persons counseled about the self-removal option.[58]

More studies are needed regarding incorporation of IUC self-removal into contraceptive counseling. That said, if a patient desires self-removal, this option may be discussed, and the provider may consider leaving device strings a bit longer to aid self-extraction.

## SUMMARY

Many contraceptives available today are more effective, safer, and better tolerated than ever before. Still, many more exciting advancements lay ahead. Although a significant investment of resources is needed to bring a new contraceptive to market, research should be encouraged. These technologies are critical to allowing individuals reproductive choice and autonomy in making this preference-sensitive decision.

## CLINICS CARE POINTS

- New available methods are members of the vaginal ring, transdermal patch, progestin-only pill, and spermicide groups.
- Updated delivery methods for IUCs, medroxyprogesterone acetate, and progestin-only implants aim to expand contraception access and safety.
- Emerging contraceptive technologies seek to improve contraceptive choice, safety, tolerability, and reproductive autonomy.

## REFERENCES

1. Daniels K, Abma JC. Current contraceptive status among women aged 15-49: United States, 2015-2017. NCHS Data Brief, No 327. Hyattsville, MD: National Center for Health Statistics; 2018.
2. Daniels K, Mosher WD. Contraceptive methods women have ever used: United States, 1982-2010. Natl Health Stat Rep 2013;(62):1–15.
3. Nelson AL. Comprehensive overview of the recently FDA-approved contraceptive vaginal ring releasing segesterone acetate and ethinylestradiol: a new year-long, patient controlled, reversible birth control method. Expert Rev Clin Pharmacol 2019;12(10):953–63.
4. Gemzell-Danielsson K, Sitruk-Ware R, Creinin MD, et al. Segesterone acetate/ethinyl estradiol 12-month contraceptive vaginal system safety evaluation. Contraception 2019;99(6):323–8.
5. Oddsson K, Leifels-Fischer B, Wiel-Masson D, et al. Superior cycle control with a contraceptive vaginal ring compared with an oral contraceptive containing 30 microg ethinylestradiol and 150 microg levonorgestrel: a randomized trial. Hum Reprod 2005;20(2):557–62.
6. Simmons KB, Kumar N, Plagianos M, et al. Effects of concurrent vaginal miconazole treatment on the absorption and exposure of Nestorone® (segesterone acetate) and ethinyl estradiol delivered from a contraceptive vaginal ring: a randomized, crossover drug-drug interaction study. Contraception 2018;97(3):270–6.
7. Kaunitz AM, Archer DF, Mishell DR Jr, et al. Safety and tolerability of a new low-dose contraceptive patch in obese and nonobese women. Am J Obstet Gynecol 2015;212(3):318.e1–8.
8. Smallwood GH, Meador ML, Lenihan JP, et al. Efficacy and safety of a transdermal contraceptive system. Obstet Gynecol 2001;98(5 Pt. 1):799–805.
9. Abrams LS, Skee DM, Natarajan J, et al. Pharmacokinetics of norelgestromin and ethinyl estradiol delivered by a contraceptive patch (Ortho Evra/Evra) under conditions of heat, humidity, and exercise. J Clin Pharmacol 2001;41(12):1301–9.
10. Archer DF, Stanczyk FZ, Rubin A, et al. Pharmacokinetics and adhesion of the Agile transdermal contraceptive patch (AG200-15) during daily exposure to

external conditions of heat, humidity and exercise. Contraception 2013;87(2): 212–9.

11. Tepper NK, Dragoman MV, Gaffield ME, et al. Nonoral combined hormonal contraceptives and thromboembolism: a systematic review. Contraception 2017; 95(2):130–9.

12. Zieman M, Guillebaud J, Weisberg E, et al. Contraceptive efficacy and cycle control with the Ortho Evra/Evra transdermal system: the analysis of pooled data. Fertil Steril 2002;77(2 Suppl 2):S13–8.

13. Archer DF, Ahrendt HJ, Drouin D. Drospirenone-only oral contraceptive: results from a multicenter noncomparative trial of efficacy, safety and tolerability. Contraception 2015;92(5):439–44.

14. Duijkers IJM, Heger-Mahn D, Drouin D, et al. Maintenance of ovulation inhibition with a new progestogen-only pill containing drospirenone after scheduled 24-h delays in pill intake. Contraception 2016;93(4):303–9.

15. Krattenmacher R. Drospirenone: pharmacology and pharmacokinetics of a unique progestogen. Contraception 2000;62(1):29–38.

16. Askew I, Wells E. DMPA-SC: an emerging option to increase women's contraceptive choices. Contraception 2018;98(5):375–8.

17. Nelson AL. An overview of properties of Amphora (Acidform) contraceptive vaginal gel. Expert Opin Drug Saf 2018;17(9):935–43.

18. Thomas MA, Chappell BT, Maximos B, et al. A novel vaginal pH regulator: results from the phase 3 AMPOWER contraception clinical trial. Contracept X 2020;2: 100031.

19. Steiner MJ, Brache V, Taylor D, et al. Randomized trial to evaluate contraceptive efficacy, safety and acceptability of a two-rod contraceptive implant over 4 years in the Dominican Republic. Contracept X 2019;1:100006.

20. Creinin MD, Kaunitz AM, Darney PD, et al. The US etonogestrel implant mandatory clinical training and active monitoring programs: 6-year experience. Contraception 2017;95(2):205–10.

21. Reed S, Do Minh T, Lange JA, et al. Real world data on Nexplanon® procedure-related events: final results from the Nexplanon Observational Risk Assessment study (NORA). Contraception 2019;100(1):31–6.

22. Iwanaga J, Fox MC, Rekers H, et al. Neurovascular anatomy of the adult female medial arm in relationship to potential sites for insertion of the etonogestrel contraceptive implant. Contraception 2019;100(1):26–30.

23. Roe AH, Bartz D. Society of family planning clinical recommendations: contraception after surgical abortion. Contraception 2019;99(1):2–9.

24. Whitaker AK, Chen BA. Society of family planning guidelines: postplacental insertion of intrauterine devices. Contraception 2018;97(1):2–13.

25. Sääv I, Stephansson O, Gemzell-Danielsson K. Early versus delayed insertion of intrauterine contraception after medical abortion—a randomized controlled trial. PLoS One 2012;7(11):e48948.

26. Shimoni N, Davis A, Ramos ME, et al. Timing of copper intrauterine device insertion after medical abortion: a randomized controlled trial. Obstet Gynecol 2011; 118(3):623–8.

27. Bednarek PH, Creinin MD, Reeves MF, et al. Immediate versus delayed IUD insertion after uterine aspiration. N Engl J Med 2011;364(23):2208–17.

28. Chen BA, Reeves MF, Hayes JL, et al. Postplacental or delayed insertion of the levonorgestrel intrauterine device after vaginal delivery: a randomized controlled trial. Obstet Gynecol 2010;116(5):1079–87.

29. Burke A, Archer D, Kimble T. New and emerging female contraceptives expand options. In: Society of Family Planning annual meeting; 2020 October 7. 2020. Virtual Conference via Zoom.

30. Apter D, Zimmerman Y, Beekman L, et al. Estetrol combined with drospirenone: an oral contraceptive with high acceptability, user satisfaction, well-being and favourable body weight control. Eur J Contracept Reprod Health Care 2017;22(4): 260–7.

31. Creinin MD, Mawet M, Ledant S, et al. P44 Phase 3 clinical trial results of a new combined oral contraceptive with estetrol 15 MG and drospirenone 3 MG. Contraception 2020;102(4):291.

32. Canonico M, Oger E, Plu-Bureau G, et al. Hormone therapy and venous thromboembolism among postmenopausal women: impact of the route of estrogen administration and progestogens: the ESTHER study. Circulation 2007;115(7): 840–5.

33. Chen MJ, Creinin MD, Turok DK, et al. Dose-finding study of a 90-day contraceptive vaginal ring releasing estradiol and segesterone acetate. Contraception 2020;102(3):168–73.

34. Jensen JT, Edelman AB, Chen BA, et al. Continuous dosing of a novel contraceptive vaginal ring releasing Nestorone® and estradiol: pharmacokinetics from a dose-finding study. Contraception 2018;97(5):422–7.

35. Kumar N, Fagart J, Liere P, et al. Nestorone® as a novel progestin for nonoral contraception: structure-activity relationships and brain metabolism studies. Endocrinology 2017;158(1):170–82.

36. Brache V, Mishell DR, Lahteenmaki P, et al. Ovarian function during use of vaginal rings delivering three different doses of Nestorone. Contraception 2001;63(5): 257–61.

37. Roy M, Hazra A, Merkatz R, et al. Progesterone vaginal ring as a new contraceptive option for lactating mothers: evidence from a multicenter non-randomized comparative clinical trial in India. Contraception 2020;102(3):159–67.

38. Duijkers IJM, Klipping C, Draeger C, et al. Ovulation inhibition with a new vaginal ring containing trimegestone. Contraception 2020;102(4):237–42.

39. Brache V, Sitruk-Ware R, Williams A, et al. Effects of a novel estrogen-free, progesterone receptor modulator contraceptive vaginal ring on inhibition of ovulation, bleeding patterns and endometrium in normal women. Contraception 2012;85(5):480–8.

40. Mahase E. Uterine fibroid drug is recalled after case of liver failure requiring transplant prompts EU review. BMJ 2020;368:m1112.

41. Reeves MF, Katz BH, Canela JM, et al. A randomized comparison of a novel nitinol-frame low-dose-copper intrauterine contraceptive and a copper T380S intrauterine contraceptive. Contraception 2017;95(6):544–8.

42. Turok DK, Nelson AL, Dart C, et al. Efficacy, safety, and tolerability of a new low-dose copper and nitinol intrauterine device: phase 2 data to 36 months. Obstet Gynecol 2020;135(4):840–7.

43. Hsia JK, Creinin MD. Intrauterine contraception. Semin Reprod Med 2016;34(3): 175–82.

44. Nelson AL, Massoudi N. New developments in intrauterine device use: focus on the US. Open Access J Contracept 2016;7:127–41.

45. Li W, Terry RN, Tang J, et al. Rapidly separable microneedle patch for the sustained release of a contraceptive. Nat Biomed Eng 2019;3(3):220–9.

46. Kirtane AR, Hua T, Hayward A, et al. A once-a-month oral contraceptive. Sci Transl Med 2019;11(521):eaay2602.

47. Mofidfar M, O'Farrell L, Prausnitz MR. Pharmaceutical jewelry: earring patch for transdermal delivery of contraceptive hormone. J Control Release 2019;301: 140–5.

48. Weinrib R, Minnis A, Agot K, et al. End-users' product preference across three multipurpose prevention technology delivery forms: baseline results from young women in Kenya and South Africa. AIDS Behav 2018;22(1):133–45.

49. Friend DR, Clark JT, Kiser PF, et al. Multipurpose prevention technologies: products in development. Antivir Res 2013;(100 Suppl):S39–47.

50. Murphy DJ, Boyd P, McCoy CF, et al. Controlling levonorgestrel binding and release in a multi-purpose prevention technology vaginal ring device. J Control Release 2016;226:138–47.

51. Anderson DJ. Antibody-based contraceptive MPTS: preclinical and clinical research. National Institute of Health; 2020. Available at: https://projectreporter. nih.gov/project_info_description.cfm?aid=9933964&icde=0.

52. Baum M. Next generation multiputpose prevention technology: an intravaginal ring for HIV prevention and nonhormonal contraception. National Institute of Health; 2020. Available at: https://projectreporter.nih.gov/project_info_ description.cfm?aid=9926590&icde=0.

53. Turok D, Gero A, Simmons R, et al. O4 The levonorgestrel vs. copper intrauterine device for emergency contraception: a non-inferiority randomized controlled trial. Contraception 2020;102(4):274.

54. Thompson I, Sanders JN, Schwarz EB, et al. Copper intrauterine device placement 6-14 days after unprotected sex. Contraception 2019;100(3):219–21.

55. Asker C, Stokes-Lampard H, Beavan J, et al. What is it about intrauterine devices that women find unacceptable? Factors that make women non-users: a qualitative study. J Fam Plann Reprod Health Care 2006;32(2):89–94.

56. Amico JR, Stimmel S, Hudson S, et al. "$231 … to pull a string!!!" American IUD users' reasons for IUD self-removal: an analysis of internet forums. Contraception 2020;101(6):393–8.

57. Foster DG, Grossman D, Turok DK, et al. Interest in and experience with IUD self-removal. Contraception 2014;90(1):54–9.

58. Raifman S, Barar R, Foster D. Effect of knowledge of self-removability of intrauterine contraceptives on uptake, continuation, and satisfaction. Womens Health Issues 2018;28(1):68–74.

# Subspecialization in Obstetrics and Gynecology

## Is It Affecting the Future Availability of Women's Health Specialists?

William F. Rayburn, MD, MBA[a],*, Imam M. Xierali, PhD[b]

KEYWORDS

• Fellowship • Obstetrics and gynecology • Residency • Subspecialty • Workforce

KEY POINTS

- Obstetrics and gynecology evolved into an accredited specialty in 1930. Subspecialties began in 1972, with 5 now being accredited and 2 having focused practice designation.
- One in every 4 obstetrician-gynecologist resident graduates pursues some form of subspecialty fellowship training, compared with 1 in 12 in 20 years ago.
- The increasing numbers of fellowship programs and positions have decreased the number of resident graduates who do not immediately pursue a fellowship.
- This trend of fewer frontline women's health specialists will be magnified by a growing US population.
- Interprofessional women's health care teams, led by well-trained obstetrician-gynecologists, will be needed to address a continued need of women in accessing health care.

## INTRODUCTION

Resident education in obstetrics and gynecology encompasses essential content areas such a primary and preventive ambulatory care, obstetrics, gynecology, reproductive endocrinology, urogynecology, minimally invasive surgery, and oncology. In a period of rapid growth and medical knowledge and technologic advancement, increasingly more is expected to be learned and subspecialization seems to be more desirable as evidenced in many medical and surgical specialties.[1] Many obstetrician-gynecologists (ob-gyns) choose to not provide or practice the entire breadth of core components required for certification by the American Board of Obstetrics and Gynecology (ABOG).[1]

[a] Department of Obstetrics and Gynecology, Medical University of South Carolina, Charleston, SC, USA; [b] Department of Family and Community Medicine, University of Texas Southwestern Medical Center, Dallas, TX, USA
* Corresponding author. 1721 Atlantic Avenue, Sullivan's Island, SC 29482.
E-mail address: wrayburnmd@gmail.com

Obstet Gynecol Clin N Am 48 (2021) 737–744
https://doi.org/10.1016/j.ogc.2021.06.003
0889-8545/21/© 2021 Elsevier Inc. All rights reserved.
obgyn.theclinics.com

Progressive subspecialization occurs in response to personal professional desires and patient demands. Although subspecialization may occur over the course of a career because of personal choice, most consider fellowship training during residency and begin immediately upon graduation.[1,2] This additional subspecialty training narrows a physician's scope of practice and could limit patient access to routine, preventive health care from ob-gyns in general practice (commonly referred to as women's health specialists).

This article is intended to report the proportion of ob-gyn resident graduates who pursued subspecialty training and to determine the growth and competitiveness of those fellowships. Owing to the concern about a potential shortfall of supply relative to demand, we attempt to answer whether this additional subspecialization is affecting the availability of women's health specialists in the US population.

## EVOLUTION OF SPECIALIZATION AND SUBSPECIALIZATION

At the onset of the twentieth century, most aspiring physicians received their training in proprietary schools that offered lectures over a 1-year period. These schools were mostly non–university-based diploma mills.[3] Furthermore, few internships were available that offered staff help at hospitals. After the Flexner report in 1910, 4-year medical schools began to replace the proprietary schools, which led to a closure of half of all US medical schools.[4] By 1914, 75% to 80% of the medical school graduates commissioned in the medical corps during World War I took 1-year internships.[5]

By 1920, most physicians were general practitioners who completed 4 years at a university or proprietary school and 1 year of hospital internship. They provided most medical care in the United States until the middle of the twentieth century. There were essentially no specialists in the early twentieth century. The first residencies were established in 1927.[4,5] By the 1930s, 13 medical specialties, including obstetrics and gynecology (in 1930), were recognized. Specialty boards were established to certify specialists. Planning for the ABOG began in 1927. The ABOG was incorporated and bylaws adopted in 1930.

In 1940, about 1 in 4 US physicians were specialists; the remainder were general practitioners who performed surgery, delivered babies, and cared for all medical conditions.[5] The military recognized physicians who demonstrated some specialty expertise with or without board certification. After World War II, there was a major shift from general practice to specialization. The proportion of postgraduate training being rotating internships declined from 75% in 1959 to 21% by 1969.[4] Shortly thereafter, obstetrics and gynecology residencies became 4-year rather than 3-year training programs upon removal of rotating internships. The term internship was replaced by the designation first postgraduate year of residency.

Subspecialties in obstetrics and gynecology began to be approved by the American Board of Medical Specialties in 1972 and authorized ABOG to certify qualified candidates. Approval of subspecialty divisions was in the following chronologic order: gynecologic oncology (1972), reproductive endocrinology and infertility (1972), maternal–fetal medicine (1972), female pelvic medicine and reproductive surgery (2011), and complex family planning (2018). The American Board of Medical Specialties approved the ABOG to offer focused practice designation in pediatric and adolescent gynecology and minimally invasive gynecologic surgery in 2019.

The National Residency Match Program (NRMP) was established in 1952 to provide a fair opportunity for applicants and program directors of residencies and fellowships to consider their options in filling positions, making reasoned decisions, and having their decisions announced at a uniform time.[6] Annual data about graduates of the

Accreditation Council for Graduate Medical Education–accredited obstetrics and gynecology residency programs and the filling of fellowship programs and positions are available from the NRMP.[6] Academic years in this report came from the most recent 20-year period from 2001 to 2020.[6,7]

## TRENDS IN RESIDENCY AND FELLOWSHIP PROGRAMS AND POSITIONS

Today, most departments of obstetrics and gynecology at US medical schools have 1 or more fellowship programs. Residents are, therefore, exposed to fellows as they rotate on different subspecialty blocks. Each subspecialty division and fellowship training program defines their scope of practice, sets standards of care and practice guidelines, provides care in complex cases, serves as trusted referral sources, and advocates for evidence-based care. The resident often participates in the wide range of education and research activities and opportunities for cross-disciplinary collaborations both institutionally and nationally.

**Fig. 1** displays the number of fellowship programs and positions filled annually for each ABOG-approved subspecialty between 2001 and 2020. These programs exclude complex family planning programs because no NRMP matching data were available until 2021.[8] The increasing number of fellowship positions related to the growing number of programs. After 2002, all fellowship programs had more applicants than available positions. The average number of applicants per position remains at 1.6 (range, 1.2–1.9) per year (trendline $P = .1353$). This ratio varies slightly from one subspecialty to another and from year to year (**Fig. 2**). Approximately 1 in 4 residency graduates is now accepted into a fellowship program, compared with 1 in 12 in 2001.

The numbers of residency graduates per year who pursued ABOG-approved fellowships or not are shown in **Fig. 3**. The increasing number of total residency graduates was offset by the number of all fellowship positions filled. The annual number of graduates not pursuing fellowship training remained constant at 989 ±37.1. As shown in **Fig. 4**, the ratio of residency graduates who did not pursue fellowship training per 100,000 adult women decreased gradually from 0.95 in 2001 to 0.75 in 2020. Stated differently, for each graduating resident not pursing a fellowship, there were 105,544 adult females in 2001 and 133,857 in 2020.

Other postgraduate training options are available to residency graduates. These include non–ABOG-approved fellowships in global women's health, reproductive infectious disease, and hospitalists. Global women's health is no longer an active program at ACOG. There are few fellowship programs for those seeking formal training as ob-gyn hospitalists, although the field is growing and involves inpatient care, predominantly in labor and delivery (https://www.sogh.org).

Regardless of subspecialty, each fellowship program is intended to develop leaders and improve care through advanced clinical, research, and education training. **Table 1** lists the years of training and whether the match is part of the NRMP for each subspecialty fellowship. Most programs accept 1 fellow per year, although this number may vary from year to year according to program size and funding. A description of each type of fellowship is beyond the scope of this article, but websites for each organization are provided in the table for additional information.

## ADJUSTING TO DECREASED ACCESSIBILITY OF WOMEN'S HEALTH SPECIALISTS

The Accreditation Council for Graduate Medical Education, NRMP, and US census data for the past 20 years demonstrate a clear trend toward a decreased accessibility of resident graduates who do not pursue fellowships (women's health specialists). We anticipate that this trend will continue as costly residency positions continue to not

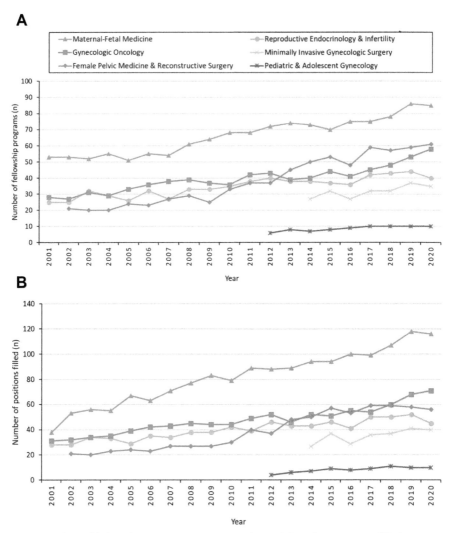

**Fig. 1.** Number of fellowship programs per year (*A*) and fellowship positions filled per year (*B*) for each ABOG-approved subspecialty, 2001 to 2020 (Note: Complex family planning fellowships were not included, because the NRMP data were unavailable until 2021).

expand significantly, all fellowship positions either expand or remain competitive, and the US population growth continues.[9]

This article is not intended to be critical about the need for subspecialty training. Subspecialists will advance select women's health care by improved diagnostic and surgical skills with potentially less morbidity. Care should improve as more subspecialists are available for consultation and either comanagement or management of complex medical and surgical cases. It is highly doubtful that subspecialists will assume the same roles as frontline women's health specialists. Some surgical subspecialists are inclined to perform a greater proportion of the decreasing number of inpatient gynecologic surgeries.[9] However, we suspect that maternal–fetal medicine

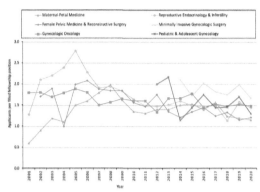

**Fig. 2.** Ratio of total applicants to fellowship positions for each ABOG-approved subspecialty, 2001 to 2020.

physicians are unlikely to perform more deliveries, especially for patients with uncomplicated pregnancies. The numbers and roles of ob-gyn hospitalists will likely expand.[10]

Findings from this report do raise concerns about the future accessibility of women's health specialists to address the general health needs of adult women. Innovations with strategic initiatives about their new roles and responsibilities as frontline ob-gyns will be necessary. Leading collaborative teams with advanced practice nonphysician clinicians (eg, nurse practitioners, certified nurse midwifes, physician assistants) and more cross-disciplinary collaboration with adult primary care providers will be necessary.[11] Frontline ob-gyns will likely engage in more general obstetrics care and less gynecologic surgery.[11,12] Furthermore, different models of care will remain necessary to address underserved communities in urban and nonurban settings.

Interprofessional collaboration in women's health care and the role of the ob-gyn has been recently summarized.[11] A goal of interprofessional collaboration is to reach the highest level of performance improvement. Through interprofessional communication and teamwork, individual providers can better understand the importance of their unique knowledge and skill set and perhaps provide an improved health care experience for patients. A future model of improvement must include not only women's

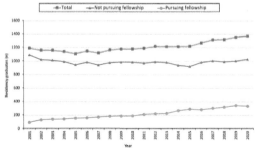

**Fig. 3.** Numbers of ob-gyn resident graduates who either pursued ABOG-approved fellowships or not, 2001 to 2020.

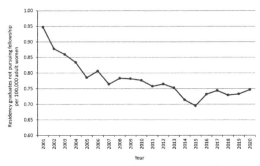

**Fig. 4.** Number of resident graduates who did not pursue fellowships per 100,000 adult women in the United States, 2001 to 2020.

health care delivery but also health system redesign (eg, practice networks, electronic health records, efficiencies, and cost effectiveness).

To be valued, interprofessional women's health teams require time and encouragement to develop, implement, and sustain programs to evaluate and recommend improvements to delivering care. This direction requires educating providers to endorse workplace learning activities such as quality improvement projects and patient safety rounds.[12,13] This generation of practitioners can oversee, advise, and ensure that other health care professionals overcome or minimize any barriers to learning within teams and that all team members display competencies in the workplace.[12]

Much of what has been recommended in the workplace is related to events in the hospital, especially in the labor and delivery unit, surgical suite, and postoperative or postpartum ward. Interprofessional collaboration in the clinic and community seems to be less obvious and perhaps more difficult to examine and measure. Obstetrics and gynecology is moving more toward ambulatory care with more interest in avoiding a nonobstetric hospital admission, emergency department referral, or inpatient surgery.[14] Outpatient consultations seem to be more common between those in women's health specialists and subspecialists. Furthermore, many adult women seek their care from primary care physicians (family physicians, general internists) and advanced practitioners, so open communication with frontline ob-gyns remains essential.

Moving forward, investment in continuing collaboration in women's health must be based on interprofessional evidence, which is accumulating. Future research can focus on addressing gaps relating to interprofessional cost–benefit analyses, organizational practice (eg, avoiding duplication, avoiding hospitalization, reducing length of patient stays and unnecessary readmissions), differences in delivering inpatient and outpatient care, and measured improvements to women's health care.

Finally, the well-being of women's health specialists has not received much attention until recently. Instead, the emphasis has been on the actions and outcomes of individual women's health providers, but stressors from health systems affects the fit and function of ob-gyns whose actions help define the effectiveness of the systems themselves. Attention about burnout (its prevalence, identification, prevention, and reversal) of ob-gyns within the system must continue.[15] A gentler, more comprehensive approach to help these frontline practitioners can decrease or reconcile stressors relating to individual and collective competencies, interactive workplace learning, and improvement in outcomes-led performances.

**Table 1**
**Fellowship training options for applicants completing an Accreditation Council for Graduate Medical Education–accredited residency in obstetrics and gynecology**

| Subspecialty | NRMP | Training Period (years) | Additional Information |
|---|---|---|---|
| Complex family planning | Yes | 2 | http://www.sfp.org |
| Female pelvic medicine and reconstructive surgery | Yes | 3 | http://www.augs.org |
| Global women's health | No | 2 | http://www.acog.org/en/ GobalWomen'sHealth/ |
| Gynecologic oncology | Yes | 3–4 | http://www.sgo.org |
| Maternal–fetal medicine | Yes | 3 | http://www.smfm.org |
| Minimally invasive gynecologic surgery | Yes | 2 | http://www.aagl.com |
| Pediatric and adolescent gynecology | Yes | 2 | http://www.naspag.org |
| Reproductive endocrinology and infertility | Yes | 3 | http://www.socrei.org |
| Reproductive infectious disease | No | 1–3 | http://www.idsog.org |

## DISCLOSURE

The authors have no financial disclosures or conflict of interest to report.

## REFERENCES

1. Rayburn WF, Gant NF, Gilstrap LC, et al. Pursuit of accredited subspecialties by graduating residents in obstetrics and gynecology, 2000-2012. Obstet Gynecol 2012;120(3):619–25.
2. Traylor J, Friedman J, Runge M, et al. Factors that influence applicants pursuing a fellowship in minimally invasive gynecologic surgery. J Minim Invasive Gynecol 2020;27:1070–5.
3. Curran JA. Internships and residencies: historical backgrounds and current trends. J Med Educ 1959;34:873–84.
4. Beck AH. The Flexner report and the standardization of American medical education. JAMA 2004;291:2139–40.
5. Starr P. The social transformation of American medicine. New York: Basic Books; 1982.
6. National Residency Matching Program. Results and data specialties matching service 2020 appointment year. Available at: https://mk0nrmp3oyqui6wqfm. kinstacdn.com/wp-content/uploads/2020/02/Results-and-Data-SMS-2020.pdf. Accessed January 31, 2021.
7. National Residency Matching Program. Obstetrics and gynecology match. Available at: http://www.nrmp.org/fellowships/obstetricsgynecology-match. Accessed January 21, 2021.
8. Schreiber C, Madden T. Complex family planning: a newly accredited, landmark fellowship. Contraception 2021;103:1–2.
9. Stonehocker J, Muruth J, Rayburn W. Is there a shortage of obstetrician-gynecologists? Obstet Gynecol Clin North Am 2017;44:121–32.

10. American College of Obstetricians and Gynecologists Committee Opinion. The obstetric and gynecologic hospitalists. No. 657, February 2016. Reaffirmed 2017.

11. Rayburn W, Jenkins C. Interprofessional collaboration in women's healthcare: collective competencies, interactive learning, and measurable input. Obstet Gynecol Clin North Am 2021;48(1):1–10.

12. Interprofessional Education Collaborative Expert Panel. Core competencies for interprofessional collaborative practice: report of an Expert Panel. Washington, DC: Interprofessional Education Collaborative; 2011.

13. Davis NL, Davis DA, Rayburn WF. Clinical faculty: taking the lead in teaching quality improvement and patient safety. Am J Obstet Gynecol 2014;211:215–6.

14. Rayburn WF, Strunk AL. Profiles about practice settings of American College of Obstetricians and Gynecologists Fellows. Obstet Gynecol 2013;122:1295–8.

15. Smith R, Rayburn W. Burnout in obstetrician-gynecologists. its prevalence, identification, prevention, and reversal. Obstet Gynecol Clin North Am 2021;48(1): 231–45.

# The Future of Fetal Surgery

Eric Bergh, MD[a],*, Cara Buskmiller, MD[b], Anthony Johnson, MD[a]

## KEYWORDS

• Fetal therapy • Fetal surgery • Fetal intervention • In utero • Fetal anomalies

## KEY POINTS

• Advances in both medical and in-utero surgical techniques have allowed for the diagnosis and treatment of fetal disorders.
• In the near-future fetal surgery will see improvements in both non-invasive and minimally invasive surgical techniques.
• In the more distant future, "ex-utero", cell-based and gene therapies may be developed to successfully treat an expanded list of fetal disorders.

## INTRODUCTION

Fetal surgery is a unique and controversial field in which multidisciplinary teams attempt the unimaginable: the application of both life-saving and life-altering therapies to the unborn patient with congenital anomalies. For the past several decades, the field has seen significant technological progress, both in fetal diagnosis and surgical approach. With improved ability to diagnose fetal conditions, the number of potential candidates for fetal surgery has risen, whereas the threshold for intervention has decreased, particularly as the morbidity associated with minimally invasive techniques continues to improve. In this article, we review some of the major innovative changes that are likely to shape the field in both the near and distant future.

At present, the field of fetal surgery is restricted predominantly to invasive procedures designed to correct or to ameliorate underlying congenital anomalies before birth. This paradigm is likely to continue into the near future, with the most visible changes occurring in the continued modification and adoption of minimally invasive surgical techniques. However, the field sits on the precipice of a major technological revolution, and breakthroughs in the fields of fetal membrane repair, robotic surgery, gene and stem cell therapy, and systems of ex utero fetal support may fundamentally change the field of fetal surgery in the more distant future.

[a] Department of Obstetrics and Gynecology, The Fetal Center at Children's Memorial Hermann Hospital, University of Texas Health Science Center, McGovern Medical School, 6410 Fannin Street, Suite 700, Houston, TX 77030, USA; [b] Maternal Fetal Medicine, Department of Obstetrics and Gynecology, University of Texas Health Science Center, McGovern Medical School, 6410 Fannin Street, Suite 700, Houston, TX 77030, USA
* Corresponding author.
E-mail address: eric.p.bergh@uth.tmc.edu
Twitter: @ericberghMD (E.B.); @CaraBuskmiller (C.B.)

Obstet Gynecol Clin N Am 48 (2021) 745–758
https://doi.org/10.1016/j.ogc.2021.06.004
0889-8545/21/Published by Elsevier Inc.
obgyn.theclinics.com

## HISTORY

The original impetus behind the development of fetal surgery was to intervene on behalf of the fetus afflicted with an otherwise life-threatening condition. The first such fetal treatments were described by Liley,[1] with the development of intrauterine transfusion, albeit via imprecise methods. Lacking modern-day ultrasound, both the diagnosis and treatment of alloimmunization relied on blind amniocentesis and amniogram-guided needle-based transfusion. With the development of ultrasound, fetal MRI, genetic diagnosis, and diagnostic fetoscopy, came the ability to more precisely diagnose fetal anomalies, to understand their natural progression during pregnancy, and to identify which anomalies might ultimately be amenable to more invasive, life-saving procedures.[2–4] Spurred on by the successful completion of the first open fetal surgery for obstructive uropathy in 1981 by Dr Michael Harrison,[5] the field of fetal surgery expanded to include treatment of additional life-threatening malformations such as congenital diaphragmatic hernia and congenital cystic adenomatoid malformation.[6] As surgical teams gained experience and procedure morbidity decreased, open fetal surgery has been extended to non–life-threatening conditions such as fetal myelomeningocele. Over time, the field of fetal surgery, initially dominated by a loose collection of global researchers publishing case reports and retrospective analyses, developed into an established surgical subspecialty with a governing society, the International Fetal Medicine Surgical Society (IFMSS),[7] and multiple randomized clinical trials[8–10]; the landmark Management of Myelomeningocele Study (MOMS) being the first to demonstrate fetal benefit from a surgical intervention in a non–life-threatening condition.[10]

Modern-day fetal surgery can be defined by several different surgical approaches to treat a variety of fetal conditions. In order of invasiveness, these include open fetal surgery, ex utero intrapartum treatment (EXIT), minimally invasive fetal surgery, and ultrasound-guided procedures.[11] The technique of choice depends on both the fetal condition and the experience of the surgical team. Many fetal diseases that were once treated via open fetal surgery are now candidates for minimally invasive fetoscopic and needle-based interventions. Examples include the treatment of fetal myelomeningocele, fetal lung lesions, and sacrococcygeal teratoma. This is perhaps the first major change in fetal surgery that will be witnessed in the near future. Although open fetal surgery, the pioneering technique that established the field, will not be abandoned entirely, its role in the future will likely diminish.[12,13] Techniques using smaller equipment, shorter operating times, and less fetal and maternal anesthesia will be adopted and optimized in favor of open surgery, which is often plagued by increased rates of preterm birth,[14] and significant maternal morbidity including implications on mode of delivery in the index pregnancy and risk to future pregnancies.[15]

Not only has the field matured from a technical perspective, but the fetal surgery community has also developed an ethical framework in which to consider the fetal patient as part of the maternal-fetal dyad. At the heart of every decision in fetal surgery is the optimization of the delicate balance between benefit to the fetus and risk to the mother. To this end, the modern fetal surgery center is typically composed of a multidisciplinary team of clinicians, researchers, geneticists, ethicists, and ancillary support staff. With the understanding that both the fetus and the mother are interdependent, decisions to offer intervention are typically based on several requirements including, but not limited to, the following:

- The need for a complete understanding of the natural history of the fetal disease with simple structural defects suitable for in utero treatment
- There should be significant hope for benefit with prenatal intervention beyond postnatal therapies

- Procedures should be performed only by a skilled multidisciplinary team
- Families must undergo full counseling on risks and benefits of the procedure[7,16,17]

In this context, this article reviews the technologies that are likely to make a large future impact on the field and may force fetal surgery teams to reconsider some of the original tenets outlined previously. With improved instrumentation and the introduction of robotics, surgeons may attempt more complex in utero repairs with minimal risk to the mother or pregnancy. The availability of gene and stem cell therapy will challenge the notion that genetic diseases are untreatable or not candidates for in utero therapy. Finally, the risk of preterm birth may become negligible if the alternative, delivery and ex utero support in an artificial womb, is optimized. These breakthrough and futuristic technologies offer a new perspective on the role for fetal surgery and will continue to change how we bring both life-saving and life-altering therapies to the fetus.

## SURGICAL REPAIR

Two major changes in the surgical method and approach to fetal surgery are on the horizon. In the near future, solving the problem of membrane injury and membrane separation during minimally invasive surgery will be a major leap forward in reducing the morbidity associated with in utero treatment of fetal diseases. In the much more distant future, application of novel robotic-based surgical techniques promises to improve complex in utero repairs.

### Membrane Repair

Minimally invasive fetal surgery has broad applications to different complex fetal disorders. There are more than 1000 fetal surgical procedures per year performed in the United States (NAFTNet.org), of which most are completed via fetoscopy. Currently, fetoscopic laser photocoagulation (FLP) of placental anastomoses in twin pregnancies complicated by twin-twin transfusion syndrome (TTTS) is one of the most common fetal surgical procedures. More recently, fetoscopy has been embraced by many groups for the repair of fetal myelomeningocele.[15]

A significant challenge and major opportunity for advancement in the field of minimally invasive fetal surgery is the complicated issue of fetal membrane injury and subsequent preterm birth. In patients undergoing fetoscopic treatment of TTTS, preterm premature rupture of membranes (PPROM) occurs in 35% of patients and shortens the pregnancy by 3 to 4 weeks of gestation.[18–20] The biological reasons for increased rates of PPROM after fetoscopy are (1) the nonhealing nature of the fetal membranes,[21,22] and (2) chorioamnion separation (CAS), which occurs when the fetal membranes detach from the uterine wall.[23] Application of significant external forces to the amniotic membrane during minimally invasive entry into the uterine cavity may translate into shearing forces, driving the separation of the amniotic membrane from the uterine wall, and thus creating a potential extra-amniotic space through which amniotic fluid may efflux. Manipulation of current straight-stick minimally invasive surgical instruments places leverage at the sight of insertion, leading to extension and enlargement of the original defect and subsequent PPROM.[24] In combination, PPROM and CAS increase the risk for intrauterine infection, preterm birth and abruption.[23] Due to the nonregenerative nature of fetal membranes, the surgical defect persists, jeopardizing the pregnancy throughout the remainder of gestation.

The inability to successfully gain access to the in utero environment percutaneously without causing major disruption of the fetal membranes continues to be both the Achilles heel of fetal surgery and a major area of research.

In cases of fetoscopy performed through a maternal laparotomy, direct access to the uterus affords the fetal surgeon the ability to place anchoring sutures at the site of trocar insertion. The technique for open fetoscopic spina bifida repair after laparotomy has shown significant promise due to the ability to effectively anchor the membranes to the uterine wall. The technique involves first exposing the uterus via laparotomy and then using ultrasound to guide placement of anchoring sutures in the membranes and myometrium with subsequent intrauterine placement of multiple fetoscopic trocars. Among 10 patients in whom this standardized technique was performed, Belfort and colleagues[25] have reported only a single case of PPROM at 34 weeks with delivery at term (39 weeks). A similar technique has been used in FLP for TTTS using a mini-laparotomy.[26] A major drawback to this technique is the invasive approach and the requirement for general anesthesia.

With this is mind, there is a critical need for novel techniques to percutaneously close fetoscopic defects in the fetal membranes. This will ultimately revolutionize fetal surgery, prolonging pregnancy and minimizing risk to both mother and fetus, and allowing for the continued development of minimally invasive and robotic techniques. There have been several attempts to develop a method to stabilize and/or repair membrane defects at the time of fetoscopy; however, to date, there are no known interventions that would reduce the risk of PPROM and CAS after percutaneous fetoscopy. Previous efforts to reduce the rates of PPROM in fetoscopy have focused on the application of surgical plugs and underwater sealant materials.[27–30] Specific challenges in this approach involve accurate application of the sealant, localized at the site of the defect, as well as the safety profile and duration of the bio-synthetic polymers. The only in utero human clinical data to date suggests that placement of a chorioamniotic collagen plug does not reduce the incidence of PPROM in patients undergoing fetoscopy for TTTS.[31] Additional studies have identified "mussel-like" glues as a potential candidate for safe and durable membrane sealing, although in vivo large animal tests have not been published and it is questionable how well such a sealant will be deployed in an aqueous environment.[32–34] One group has made recent headway toward solving this problem with the development of an ex vivo umbrellalike device with the ability to deliver underwater glue to a membrane defect.[35] Another group has recently published on the development of an ex vivo semirigid biocompatible silicone patch coated with bioadhesive.[36] Neither of these innovative devices has been tested clinically, although both show promise as nontoxic, durable, and potentially elastic adhesives. Further in vivo development of these approaches may ultimately lead to improved outcomes, although it may also be the case that the ideal approach to this problem has yet to be discovered. Potentially an in utero/fetoscopic suture-based approach, similar to anchoring sutures placed at the time of open fetoscopy, might be a safe and effective method of membrane repair.

### Robotic Surgery

A major limitation to the current method of fetoscopic surgery is the reliance on multiple fetoscopic ports and straight-stick instrumentation initially designed for pediatric and adult laparoscopy to accomplish complex in utero repairs. Importantly, the manipulation and surgical repair of fetal defects requires a degree of precision and tissue manipulation not easily attained with current fetoscopic surgical instrumentation. Future advances in robotic surgery have the potential to address this problem.

Robotic surgery in adult and pediatric medicine has transformed the operating room and pushed the field of minimally invasive surgery to a new frontier. As opposed to straight-stick laparoscopy, the surgical robot allows for articulated manipulation of delicate tissues with added motion stabilization, 3-dimensional optics, as well as improved surgeon comfort and the possibility of remote/telesurgery. The need for additional training and specialized equipment has somewhat limited the use of the surgical robot, as has its size and current docking requirements. However, with continued improvements and further device miniaturization, there has been rapid adoption of the technology outside of fetal surgery.

Presently, the application of robotics to fetal surgery is experimental, with published reports limited to animal models.[37–39] However, for the same reasons many adult and pediatric procedures have adopted robotic techniques, the emergency of "febotics" for in utero fetal procedures may be considered a natural progression.[40] The improved dexterity and field of view attained with robotics will be a major leap forward in the surgical treatment of fetal diseases, where spaces are small and often inaccessible, and the fetal tissue at midgestation is particularly friable and delicate. Furthermore, articulated movements allow for a precise surgical repair that is typically only achieved during open fetal surgery.

Previous application of robotic surgical technology to the animal model has led to several observations. Unique to fetal surgery is the decision to use either a laparotomy approach versus a percutaneous approach. In the lamb model, Knight and colleagues[41] found that the support of the abdominal wall in the percutaneous approach led to less fluid leakage than with open hysterotomy; however, the rate of membrane separation was exceedingly high (86%) without a percutaneous method to anchor or patch the multiple membrane defects. Kohl and colleagues[38] noted a significant increase in the operative setup time with a robotic approach. However, performing a lumbosacral repair in fetal sheep was far more ergonomic at a robotic console and allowed significantly improved visualization and tissue manipulation over traditional straight-stick manual fetoscopic closure. In one case, abnormal fetal positioning forced the team to abandon the robotic technique, as the robotic arms could not adjust to the acute angles of approach.[38] This may result from the fact that the evolution of robotic devices has not yet reached the small scale necessary to perform within the confines of the limited intrauterine space. Future devices will need strategies to effectively manipulate and position the fetus while working within a limited operative space.

An additional potential benefit to robotic surgery will be the ability to allow experienced surgeons to work remotely and to potentially guide local teams through complex repairs at distant sites. The rise of telemedicine in fetal surgery will allow for the further consolidation of medical experience into centers of excellence with the ability to work remotely at great distances, potentially bringing critical expertise to underserved areas.

At present, the leap to robotic fetal surgery remains on the surgical horizon; however, with continued miniaturization of instrumentation, the field is likely to see the application of robotics to complex repairs such as fetal myelomeningocele as well as defects for which we currently have no in utero surgical repair, such as fetal gastroschisis or congenital diaphragmatic hernia. Looking toward the distant future, the development of untethered micro-robotic systems, powered by external or onboard energy sources, may be the ultimate solution to surgical repair and tissue manipulation in the fetus.[40,42,43] The development of micro-robots with onboard cameras and self-assembling components may someday allow for improved navigation within an aqueous in utero environment. Such theoretic and futuristic devices may one day perform tissue repair or deliver targeted therapeutics such as gene or stem cell therapies to the fetus with minimal risk to the mother or the pregnancy.[44]

## STEM CELL AND GENE THERAPY

The future of fetal therapy also promises nonsurgical therapies that add to or change the genotype of the fetus. These therapies redirect fetal organ development, occasionally in cooperation with surgical interventions.

Fetal medicine has seen several decades of improvements in prenatal genetic diagnosis, from chromosomal microarray to cell-free fetal DNA and its growing applications. Along with these diagnostic abilities, techniques have developed to modify genetic expression and to alter the course of disease, although most still demand further clinical investigation. In the near and distant future, the field of fetal intervention will see further development of in utero stem cell and gene therapies for the treatment of congenital diseases.

### Stem Cell Therapy

Stem cell therapy has 2 main applications to fetal conditions. Stem cells harvested from an allogeneic donor may be grafted into the developing fetus, with the purpose of replacing fetal cell lines and reversing disease before the accumulation of significant damage. Alternatively, fetal stem cells have the potential to serve as external tissue grafts in the surgical repair of fetal anatomic malformations. Both are avenues by which fetal disease may be treated with these unique populations of multipotent cells.

The early fetus has several properties that make it particularly suitable to treatment with stem cells in general. These include an immature immune system, small physical size, multiple large populations of undifferentiated cells, and the potential of those populations to proliferate rapidly.[45] Furthermore, targeting the developing fetus allows for potential treatment before the onset of disease.

The idea of purposefully investing a fetus with a duplicate, allogeneic line of stem cells arose after twin cows were found to have spontaneously chimeric bone marrow lines,[46] and this proved to be inducible using in utero hematopoietic stem cell transplantation.[47–49] Here, the teachable immune system of the fetus allows a new line of stem cells to replace an existing line, which can cure certain congenital conditions. The fetal immune system can acquire tolerance to the donor's antigens without the burden of immunosuppression, because of its immature state.[50,51]

Hematopoietic stem cell therapy has been successful in humans in cases of congenital absence of an entire cell line, as in X-linked severe combined immunodeficiency.[52–54] However, hematopoietic stem cell transplants do not work as well when they attempt to replace a barely functional or functional cell line, such as in sickle cell disease. In contrast, mesenchymal cells, which are less immunogenic, have seen some success in the in utero treatment of Gaucher disease[55,56] and osteogenesis imperfecta.[57–59]

The other widely studied use of stem cell therapy in human fetuses is use of congenic stem cells from the fetus itself in proposed fetal tissue engineering. Briefly, this involves harvesting mesenchymal cells from amniotic fluid or other fetal tissue and culturing these cells to create a tissue graft that can then be implanted to correct anatomic defects such as myelomeningocele,[60] congenital diaphragmatic hernia,[61] or trachea-esophageal fistula.[62,63] This approach, combined with fetal or pediatric surgery, offers grafts of greater longevity with potentially better long-term outcomes. At this point, all applications for fetal tissue engineering are in animal models.

Currently, both of these types of stem cell therapy are considered experimental, and there are several important limitations to consider. When a fetus's own stem cells are used as material for stem cell transplantation, there are no immune barriers,[64] but when an allogeneic (donor) cell population is used, the fetus does not always accept the donor's new antigens: the immune system is not always perfectly "teachable."[65] Finally, there is a *maternal* barrier via placental[66] and even postnatal[67] transfer of antibodies and T cells.

These barriers still require study, but have not completely inhibited the success of allogeneic techniques. Both allogeneic transplants for missing cell lines and congenic tissue grafts are promising therapies that complement fetal surgery and almost certainly have a place in the near future of fetal therapy.

### Gene Therapy

The rationale behind gene therapy is similar to fetal cell transplantation: in the small fetal recipient, an efficient dose and teachable immune system can stop a disease process before it affects further development. Gene therapy is typically carried out with a viral vector containing the gene to be transplanted. Although nonviral vector approaches exist, most animal models and early human studies of gene therapy have implemented adenoviruslike capsids.

When applied to the early embryo, intraamniotic administration of gene therapy allows for whole-body penetration via all 3 exposed germ layers during embryologic folding.[68,69] Later in gestation, fetal breathing allows inhalation therapy targeted to pulmonary epithelium in a murine model.[70] Different viral vectors can be exploited for the human tissues they naturally seek out, which allows targeted therapy to multiple tissues.

As of yet, success in curing fetal disease has been limited to animal models of disorders such as muscle developmental disorders, hemophilia, and Wilson disease.[71–73] Gene therapy has been used in adult humans with hemophilia, but is not yet considered standard of care.[74]

Fetal gene therapy offers several advantages over postnatal therapy. First, adults carry condition-specific antibodies to many protein products they do not express. For example, pediatric and adult patients with cystic fibrosis have antibodies against cystic fibrosis transmembrane conductance regulator products, which threaten the therapeutic potential of any gene therapy applied postnatally.[75] Although it is not clear whether fetuses have condition-specific antibodies, their antibody development is typically less mature and production of such antibodies declines with gene therapy itself.[76]

Second, fetal patients have had no exposure to viral vectors, whereas neonates quickly encounter adenovirus and other viruses after birth and create antibodies to them. As a result, within the confines of the protected uterine environment, the fetal immune system can learn tolerance to the viral vector, allowing for repeated postnatal injection without an immune response.[77,78] These 2 advantages mean viral vector gene therapy is inviting and feasible for select congenital conditions, and is very likely part of the future of fetal therapy for single-gene disorders.

### CRISPR/Cas9

The use of the CRISPR/CAS9 pathway to splice and replace sequences of the human genome offers another possibility for repair of single-gene disorders.[79] Here, the greatest advantage the fetus offers is rapidly proliferating cells (rather than small size or immune immaturity). The rapidly proliferating nature of fetal tissue means that cells with a spliced and repaired genome can quickly build up a population, produce normal gene products, educate the immune system, and halt disease effects.[79] Mouse models of muscular dystrophy[80] and enzyme defects[81] have successfully eliminated disease and incorporated functional DNA sequences into their host.

The risks of CRISPR/CAS9 are still poorly characterized and largely theoretic. Risks may include insertional mutagenesis, disruption of other normal processes, and unknown effects of altering the germline.[45] Despite its newness, CRISR/Cas9 has been successfully used in adults with sickle cell disease and beta thalassemia using autologous bone marrow.

As CRISPR/Cas9, viral vector gene therapy, and stem cell transplants continue to develop into clinical solutions, they will undoubtedly play an important role in the future treatment of fetal diseases.

## ARTIFICIAL WOMB

Premature birth secondary to invasive fetal therapy continues to be a major source of neonatal morbidity. Research directed toward the development of an ex vivo uterine environment therapy, otherwise known as the "artificial womb," aims to reduce the morbidity associated with peri-viable and preterm delivery. The driving force behind such research is the lack of significant improvements in outcomes for children born at the border of viability (21–24 weeks' gestation),[82] as the most severe morbidity occurs in children born within this age group.[83–87]

The womb has traditionally been seen as the best intensive care unit for the developing fetus. However, the artificial placenta aims to challenge that idea, and to restructure our ideas about preterm birth, not as a possible complication, but rather as a possible treatment option. In theory, some in utero therapies, such as myelomeningocele repair, congenital diaphragmatic hernia repair, or fetal gene therapy, could be offered after safe delivery and transition of a premature fetus to an artificial womb system.

A central idea behind the development of the artificial womb is the ability to maintain a normal fetal physiology in the newly delivered premature infant. This is in opposition to traditional and current practice of treating the fetus as a gas-ventilated neonate. Rather, the artificial womb avoids gas-based ventilation and maintains patency of the fetal circulatory system, that is, prevention of closure of fetal shunts.[82]

At the most basic level, components of the artificial placenta design include (1) timed surgical delivery, (2) catheterization of the fetal circulatory system and attachment to a membrane oxygenator circuit, and (3) transfer of the fetus into a sterile amniotic fluid bath. Both invasive (serologic) and noninvasive (ultrasound) methods are used to assess fetal status and to guide any fine-tuning of circuit parameters.

A major challenge in the development of the artificial womb has been the ability to successfully maintain an extremely premature fetus on extracorporeal circulation. This has been, in part, due to the fragility of the fetal cardiopulmonary system, the inability to safely provide pulmonary gas exchange without significant damage to the respiratory system, dependence on systems of anticoagulation within the fetal circuit, and the high susceptibility to infection at this gestational age.[82] Recently, several groups have reported successes in maintaining fetal lambs delivered at 95 days gestational age (dGA) and 105 to 113 dGA, approximately equivalent to 21 to 24 weeks' gestation on ex utero environments.[82,88] Unique to both approaches is the strict reliance on umbilical cord catheterization techniques (avoiding usage of pulmonary ventilation and carotid artery or jugular vein catheterization), using a pumpless low-resistance circuit, and the development of a closed sterile amniotic housing unit. Compared with age-matched in utero controls, fetal lambs show similar growth, lung maturation, and brain histology, although long-term assessment of neurologic function has not been assessed.[82,88]

While promising, several major challenges preclude immediate application of this experimental technology to a human model. Questions remain as to (1) the safety of prolonged usage of corticosteroids in the treatment of fetal hypotension, (2) prolonged exposure to antibiotic therapy, (3) exposure to noxious stimuli in an artificial uterine environment, and (4) the ability to prevent fetal intracranial hemorrhage and adverse long-term neurologic sequelae.[89] Furthermore, the application of this technology has several logistic and ethical limitations. Successful transition of the preterm fetus to the ex utero environment requires a scheduled surgical delivery via EXIT with classic cesarean section, which has significant maternal risk both in the index pregnancy and for any future pregnancy. Also, it is unclear whether children born vaginally or in the setting of preterm labor or intrauterine infection could be successfully transitioned to extracorporeal circulation due to the need for a coordinated delivery and the high risk for sepsis.[89,90] Finally, questions remain as to who would bear ultimate responsibility for the medical decision making and treatment of a fetus on ex utero support.[89]

The future of the artificial placenta will depend on the ability to mitigate the preceding risks, particularly with respect to fetal intracranial hemorrhage and risk for infection at the limits of viability, and then to transition this technology to a human model. In the future, the development of an optimized ex utero support system may be an important safety net for patients who choose to undergo fetal surgery and who remain at continued risk for delivery at the extremes of prematurity.

## SUMMARY

In this article, we have outlined how several breakthroughs in technology will ultimately change the field of fetal surgery. The future of the field will be defined by a trend toward the adoption of minimally invasive techniques, with improved morbidity profiles for both mother and fetus. Conditions that are currently deemed untreatable during pregnancy may ultimately have an in utero treatment either via precision robotic-assisted surgery, or via stem cell or gene therapy. With the further development of the artificial womb, the entire paradigm of in utero versus ex utero surgery will change, and may spur the development of yet another niche subspecialized field in ex utero fetal support and therapy. Although it may be years before any of these changes come to fruition, the field is poised to embrace new and novel techniques for the treatment of fetal conditions.

## CLINICS CARE POINTS

- The most common complication in minimally invasive fetoscopy is insult to the fetal membranes resulting in preterm rupture and early delivery. Future methods to reduce this complication will expand the ability to safely perform fetal interventions.
- Continued improvements and minimization may lead to utilization of robotics in the surgical treatment of fetal diseases.
- Development of additional cell-based, gene-based and "ex-utero" treatments may ultimately change our approach to treatment of the fetus.

## DISCLOSURE

The authors have nothing to disclose.

## REFERENCES

1. Liley AW. The use of amniocentesis and fetal transfusion in erythroblastosis fetalis. Pediatrics 1965;35:836–47.
2. Elias S, Verp MS. Prenatal diagnosis of genetic disorders. Obstet Gynecol Annu 1983;12:79–102.

3. Gohari P, Spinelli A. Fetoscopy in the practice of perinatology and obstetrics. Obstet Gynecol Annu 1979;8:179–202.

4. Benzie RJ, Doran TA. The "fetoscope"–a new clinical tool for prenatal genetic diagnosis. Am J Obstet Gynecol 1975;121:460–4.

5. First fetal surgery survivor finally meets his doctor. 2021. Available at: https://fetus.ucsf.edu/news/first-fetal-surgery-survivor-finally-meets-his-doctor.    Accessed March 5 2021.

6. Koehler SM, Knezevich M, Wagner A. The evolution of fetal surgery. J Fetal Surg 2017;1(1):7–23.

7. Harrison MR, Filly RA, Golbus MS, et al. Fetal treatment 1982. N Engl J Med 1982; 307:1651–2.

8. Slaghekke F, Lopriore E, Lewi L, et al. Fetoscopic laser coagulation of the vascular equator versus selective coagulation for twin-to-twin transfusion syndrome: an open-label randomised controlled trial. Lancet 2014;383:2144–51.

9. Morris RK, Malin GL, Quinlan-Jones E, et al. Percutaneous vesicoamniotic shunting versus conservative management for fetal lower urinary tract obstruction (PLUTO): a randomised trial. Lancet 2013;382:1496–506.

10. Adzick NS, Thom EA, Spong CY, et al. A randomized trial of prenatal versus postnatal repair of myelomeningocele. N Engl J Med 2011;364:993–1004.

11. Farrell J, Howell LJ. An overview of surgical techniques, research trials, and future directions of fetal therapy. J Obstet Gynecol neonatal Nurs 2012;41: 419–25.

12. Flake AW. Surgery in the human fetus: the future. J Physiol 2003;547:45–51.

13. Harrison MR. Fetal surgery: trials, tribulations, and turf. J Pediatr Surg 2003;38: 275–82.

14. Deprest J, Gratacos E, Nicolaides KH, et al. Fetoscopic tracheal occlusion (FETO) for severe congenital diaphragmatic hernia: evolution of a technique and preliminary results. Ultrasound Obstet Gynecol 2004;24:121–6.

15. Sacco A, Van der Veeken L, Bagshaw E, et al. Maternal complications following open and fetoscopic fetal surgery: a systematic review and meta-analysis. Prenat Diagn 2019;39:251–68.

16. Wenstrom KD, Carr SR. Fetal surgery: principles, indications, and evidence. Obstet Gynecol 2014;124:817–35.

17. Sharma D, Tsibizova VI. Current perspective and scope of fetal therapy: part 1. J Matern Fetal Neonatal Med 2020;1–29. https://doi.org/10.1080/14767058. 2020.1839880.

18. Yamamoto M, El Murr L, Robyr R, et al. Incidence and impact of perioperative complications in 175 fetoscopy-guided laser coagulations of chorionic plate anastomoses in fetofetal transfusion syndrome before 26 weeks of gestation. Am J Obstet Gynecol 2005;193:1110–6.

19. Snowise S, Mann LK, Moise KJ Jr, et al. Preterm prelabor rupture of membranes after fetoscopic laser surgery for twin-twin transfusion syndrome. Ultrasound Obstet Gynecol 2017;49:607–11.

20. Stirnemann J, Djaafri F, Kim A, et al. Preterm premature rupture of membranes is a collateral effect of improvement in perinatal outcomes following fetoscopic coagulation of chorionic vessels for twin-twin transfusion syndrome: a retrospective observational study of 1092 cases. BJOG 2018;125:1154–62.

21. Gratacos E, Sanin-Blair J, Lewi L, et al. A histological study of fetoscopic membrane defects to document membrane healing. Placenta 2006;27:452–6.

22. Papanna R, Bebbington MW, Moise K Jr. Novel findings of iatrogenic fetal membrane defect after previous fetoscopy for twin-twin transfusion syndrome. Ultrasound Obstet Gynecol 2013;42:118–9.
23. Papanna R, Mann LK, Johnson A, et al. Chorioamnion separation as a risk for preterm premature rupture of membranes after laser therapy for twin-twin transfusion syndrome. Obstet Gynecol 2010;115:771–6.
24. Kohl T. Iatrogenic fetal membrane damage from complex fetoscopic surgery in human fetuses might not be amenable to simple closure by collagen plugs. Prenat Diagn 2008;28:876–7 [author reply: 8–80].
25. Belfort MA, Whitehead WE, Shamshirsaz AA, et al. Fetoscopic open neural tube defect repair: development and refinement of a two-port, carbon dioxide insufflation technique. Obstet Gynecol 2017;129:734–43.
26. Deprest JA, Van Schoubroeck D, Van Ballaer PP, et al. Alternative technique for Nd:YAG laser coagulation in twin-to-twin transfusion syndrome with anterior placenta. Ultrasound Obstet Gynecol 1998;11:347–52.
27. Papanna R, Molina S, Moise KY, et al. Chorioamnion plugging and the risk of preterm premature rupture of membranes after laser surgery in twin-twin transfusion syndrome. Ultrasound Obstet Gynecol 2010;35:337–43.
28. Chang J, Tracy TF Jr, Carr SR, et al. Port insertion and removal techniques to minimize premature rupture of the membranes in endoscopic fetal surgery. J Pediatr Surg 2006;41:905–9.
29. Luks FI, Deprest JA, Peers KH, et al. Gelatin sponge plug to seal fetoscopy port sites: technique in ovine and primate models. Am J Obstet Gynecol 1999;181: 995–6.
30. Reddy UM, Shah SS, Nemiroff RL, et al. In vitro sealing of punctured fetal membranes: potential treatment for midtrimester premature rupture of membranes. Am J Obstet Gynecol 2001;185:1090–3.
31. Papanna R, Mann LK, Moise KY, et al. Absorbable gelatin plug does not prevent iatrogenic preterm premature rupture of membranes after fetoscopic laser surgery for twin-twin transfusion syndrome. Ultrasound Obstet Gynecol 2013;42: 456–60.
32. Bilic G, Brubaker C, Messersmith PB, et al. Injectable candidate sealants for fetal membrane repair: bonding and toxicity in vitro. Am J Obstet Gynecol 2010;202: 85.e1-9.
33. Haller CM, Buerzle W, Kivelio A, et al. Mussel-mimetic tissue adhesive for fetal membrane repair: an ex vivo evaluation. Acta Biomater 2012;8:4365–70.
34. Kivelio A, Dekoninck P, Perrini M, et al. Mussel mimetic tissue adhesive for fetal membrane repair: initial in vivo investigation in rabbits. Eur J Obstet Gynecol Reprod Biol 2013;171:240–5.
35. Devaud YR, Zuger S, Zimmermann R, et al. Minimally invasive surgical device for precise application of bioadhesives to prevent iPPROM. Fetal Diagn Ther 2019; 45:102–10.
36. Micheletti T, Eixarch E, Berdun S, et al. Ex-vivo mechanical sealing properties and toxicity of a bioadhesive patch as sealing system for fetal membrane iatrogenic defects. Sci Rep 2020;10:18608.
37. Kosa G, Jakab P, Szekely G, et al. MRI driven magnetic microswimmers. Biomed Microdevices 2012;14:165–78.
38. Kohl T, Hartlage MG, Kiehitz D, et al. Percutaneous fetoscopic patch coverage of experimental lumbosacral full-thickness skin lesions in sheep. Surg Endosc 2003; 17:1218–23.

39. Aaronson OS, Tulipan NB, Cywes R, et al. Robot-assisted endoscopic intrauterine myelomeningocele repair: a feasibility study. Pediatr Neurosurg 2002;36:85–9.
40. Berris M, Shoham M. Febotics - a marriage of fetal surgery and robotics. Comput Aided Surg 2006;11:175–80.
41. Knight CG, Lorincz A, Johnson A, et al. Robot-enhanced fetoscopic surgery. J Pediatr Surg 2004;39:1463–5.
42. Li J, Esteban-Fernandez de Avila B, Gao W, et al. Micro/nanorobots for biomedicine: delivery, surgery, sensing, and detoxification. Sci Robot 2017;2. eaam6431.
43. Boswell T. Robotic fetal surgery: the next frontier? Available at: https://link.springer.com/chapter/10.1007%2F978-3-030-57219-8_25.
44. Nikitichev DI, Shakir DI, Chadebecq F, et al. Medical-grade sterilizable target for fluid-immersed fetoscope optical distortion calibration. J Vis Exp 2017;(120):55298.
45. Witt R, MacKenzie TC, Peranteau WH. Fetal stem cell and gene therapy. Semin Fetal Neonatal Med 2017;22:410–4.
46. Owen R. Immunogenic consequences of vascular anastomoses between bovine twins. Science 1945;102:400–1.
47. Billingham RE, Brent L, Medawar PB. 'Actively acquired tolerance' of foreign cells. Nature 1953;172:603–6.
48. Fleischman RA, Mintz B. Prevention of genetic anemias in mice by microinjection of normal hematopoietic stem cells into the fetal placenta. Proc Natl Acad Sci 1979;76:5736–40.
49. Fleischman RA, Mintz B. Development of adult bone marrow stem cells in H-2-compatible and -incompatible mouse fetuses. J Exp Med 1984;159:731–45.
50. Peranteau WH, Hayashi S, Hsieh M, et al. High-level allogeneic chimerism achieved by prenatal tolerance induction and postnatal nonmyeloablative bone marrow transplantation. Blood 2002;100:2225–34.
51. Nijagal A, Derderian C, Le T, et al. Direct and indirect antigen presentation lead to deletion of donor-specific T cells after in utero hematopoietic cell transplantation in mice. Blood 2013;121:4595–602.
52. Touraine JL, Raudrant D, Royo C, et al. In-utero transplantation of stem cells in bare lymphocyte syndrome. Lancet 1989;1:1382.
53. Flake AW, Roncarolo MG, Puck JM, et al. Treatment of X-linked severe combined immunodeficiency by in utero transplantation of paternal bone marrow. N Engl J Med 1996;335:1806–10.
54. Wengler GS, Lanfranchi A, Frusca T, et al. In-utero transplantation of parental CD34 haematopoietic progenitor cells in a patient with X-linked severe combined immunodeficiency (SCIDXI). Lancet 1996;348:1484–7.
55. Tiblad E, Westgren M. Fetal stem-cell transplantation. Best Pract Res Clin Obstet Gynaecol 2008;22:189–201.
56. Weiss K, Gonzalez A, Lopez G, et al. The clinical management of Type 2 Gaucher disease. Mol Genet Metab 2015;114:110–22.
57. Le Blanc K, Gotherstrom C, Ringden O, et al. Fetal mesenchymal stem-cell engraftment in bone after in utero transplantation in a patient with severe osteogenesis imperfecta. Transplantation 2005;79:1607–14.
58. Palanki R, Peranteau WH, Mitchell MJ. Delivery technologies for in utero gene therapy. Adv Drug Deliv Rev 2020;169:51–62.
59. Gotherstrom C, Westgren M, Shaw SW, et al. Pre- and postnatal transplantation of fetal mesenchymal stem cells in osteogenesis imperfecta: a two-center experience. Stem Cells Transl Med 2014;3:255–64.

60. Galganski LA, Kumar P, Vanover MA, et al. In utero treatment of myelomeningocele with placental mesenchymal stromal cells - Selection of an optimal cell line in preparation for clinical trials. J Pediatr Surg 2020;55:1941–6.

61. Kunisaki SM, Fuchs JR, Kaviani A, et al. Diaphragmatic repair through fetal tissue engineering: a comparison between mesenchymal amniocyte- and myoblast-based constructs. J Pediatr Surg 2006;41:34–9 [discussion: -9].

62. Fuchs JR, Hannouche D, Terada S, et al. Fetal tracheal augmentation with cartilage engineered from bone marrow-derived mesenchymal progenitor cells. J Pediatr Surg 2003;38:984–7.

63. Fuchs JR, Terada S, Ochoa ER, et al. Fetal tissue engineering: in utero tracheal augmentation in an ovine model. J Pediatr Surg 2002;37:1000–6 [discussion: -6].

64. Peranteau WH, Endo M, Adibe OO, et al. Evidence for an immune barrier after in utero hematopoietic-cell transplantation. Blood 2007;109:1331–3.

65. Durkin ET, Jones KA, Rajesh D, et al. Early chimerism threshold predicts sustained engraftment and NK-cell tolerance in prenatal allogeneic chimeras. Blood 2008;112:5245–53.

66. Nijagal A, Wegorzewska M, Jarvis E, et al. Maternal T cells limit engraftment after in utero hematopoietic cell transplantation in mice. J Clin Invest 2011;121:582–92.

67. Merianos DJ, Tiblad E, Santore MT, et al. Maternal alloantibodies induce a postnatal immune response that limits engraftment following in utero hematopoietic cell transplantation in mice. J Clin Invest 2009;119(9):2590–600.

68. Stitelman DH, Brazelton T, Bora A, et al. Developmental stage determines efficiency of gene transfer to muscle satellite cells by in utero delivery of adeno-associated virus vector serotype 2/9. Mol Ther Methods Clin Dev 2014;1:14040.

69. Endo M, Henriques-Coelho T, Zoltick PW, et al. The developmental stage determines the distribution and duration of gene expression after early intra-amniotic gene transfer using lentiviral vectors. Gene Ther 2010;17:61–71.

70. Joyeux L, Danzer E, Limberis MP, et al. In utero lung gene transfer using adeno-associated viral and lentiviral vectors in mice. Hum Gene Ther Methods 2014;25: 197–205.

71. Sabatino DE, Mackenzie TC, Peranteau W, et al. Persistent expression of hF.IX after tolerance induction by in utero or neonatal administration of AAV-1-F.IX in hemophilia B mice. Mol Ther 2007;15:1677–85.

72. Roybal JL, Endo M, Radu A, et al. Early gestational gene transfer with targeted ATP7B expression in the liver improves phenotype in a murine model of Wilson's disease. Gene Ther 2012;19:1085–94.

73. Koppanati BM, Li J, Xiao X, et al. Systemic delivery of AAV8 in utero results in gene expression in diaphragm and limb muscle: treatment implications for muscle disorders. Gene Ther 2009;16:1130–7.

74. George LA, Fogarty PF. Gene therapy for hemophilia: past, present and future. Semin Hematol 2016;53:46–54.

75. Calcedo R, Griesenbach U, Dorgan DJ, et al. Self-reactive CFTR T cells in humans: implications for gene therapy. Hum Gene Ther Clin Dev 2013;24:108–15.

76. Mingozzi F, Maus MV, Hui DJ, et al. CD8+ T-cell responses to adeno-associated virus capsid in humans. Nat Med 2007;13:419–22.

77. Davey MG, Riley JS, Andrews A, et al. Induction of immune tolerance to foreign protein via adeno-associated viral vector gene transfer in mid-gestation fetal sheep. PLoS One 2017;12:e0171132.

78. Calcedo R, Morizono H, Wang L, et al. Adeno-associated virus antibody profiles in newborns, children, and adolescents. Clin Vaccin Immunol 2011;18:1586–8.

79. Maeder ML, Gersbach CA. Genome-editing technologies for gene and cell therapy. Mol Ther 2016;24:430–46.

80. Yang Y, Wang L, Bell P, et al. A dual AAV system enables the Cas9-mediated correction of a metabolic liver disease in newborn mice. Nat Biotechnol 2016; 34:334–8.

81. Tabebordbar M, Zhu K, Cheng JKW, et al. In vivo gene editing in dystrophic mouse muscle and muscle stem cells. Science 2016;351:407–11.

82. Usuda H, Watanabe S, Saito M, et al. Successful use of an artificial placenta to support extremely preterm ovine fetuses at the border of viability. Am J Obstet Gynecol 2019;221:69 e1–e17.

83. Stoll BJ, Hansen NI, Bell EF, et al. Trends in care practices, morbidity, and mortality of extremely preterm neonates, 1993-2012. JAMA 2015;314:1039–51.

84. Stoinska B, Gadzinowski J. Neurological and developmental disabilities in ELBW and VLBW: follow-up at 2 years of age. J Perinatol 2011;31:137–42.

85. Stoll BJ, Hansen NI, Bell EF, et al. Neonatal outcomes of extremely preterm infants from the NICHD Neonatal Research Network. Pediatrics 2010;126:443–56.

86. Brumbaugh JE, Hansen NI, Bell EF, et al. Outcomes of extremely preterm infants with birth weight less than 400 g. JAMA Pediatr 2019;173:434–45.

87. Anderson JG, Baer RJ, Partridge JC, et al. Survival and major morbidity of extremely preterm infants: a population-based study. Pediatrics 2016;138: e20154434.

88. Partridge EA, Davey MG, Hornick MA, et al. An extra-uterine system to physiologically support the extreme premature lamb. Nat Commun 2017;8:15112.

89. Sahoo T, Gulla KM. Artificial placenta: miles to go before I sleep. Am J Obstet Gynecol 2019;221:368–9.

90. Usuda H, Watanabe S, Saito M, et al. Successful use of an artificial placenta-based life support system to treat extremely preterm ovine fetuses compromised by intrauterine inflammation. Am J Obstet Gynecol 2020;223:755.e1–20.

# Robotic Surgery

## Advancements and Inflection Points in the Field of Gynecology

Esther S. Han, MD, MPH, Arnold P. Advincula, MD*

### KEYWORDS

- Robotic surgery • Ergonomics • Surgeon console • Haptic feedback
- Stereoscopic imaging • Hospital privileging

### KEY POINTS

- Despite previous controversies, the use of robotic surgery continues to grow and expand.
- New robotic surgery systems are entering the marketplace and will compete with the various da Vinci Surgical Systems.
- New robotic platforms on the horizon aim to improve surgeon ergonomics and provide haptic feedback.
- New robotic platforms are often smaller, modular, and more versatile than the currently available surgical systems.
- Hospital privileging for robotic surgery is highly variable and largely inadequate and must be strengthened and standardized as robotic surgery increases and new technologies enter the marketplace.

## ADVENT AND CURRENT STATUS OF ROBOTIC SURGERY IN GYNECOLOGY

One particular platform, the da Vinci Surgical System (Intuitive Surgical, Inc, Sunnyvale, CA, USA) (**Figs. 1** and **2**), has both transformed and dominated the surgical robotics marketplace globally since the public launch of its first generation in 2000. Once it gained Food and Drug Administration (FDA) approval for gynecologic surgical procedures in April 2005, the da Vinci Surgical System's utility in gynecologic surgery was quickly recognized,[1] and there has been a dramatic and steady increase in uptake. After general surgery, gynecology now performs the second highest robotic surgical volume in the United States. In 2018, approximately 265,000 gynecologic procedures were performed robotically.[2]

Columbia University Irving Medical Center, 622 West 168th Street, PH16-139, New York, NY 10032, USA
* Corresponding author.
E-mail address: aa3530@cumc.columbia.edu

Obstet Gynecol Clin N Am 48 (2021) 759–776
https://doi.org/10.1016/j.ogc.2021.07.004
0889-8545/21/© 2021 Elsevier Inc. All rights reserved.

obgyn.theclinics.com

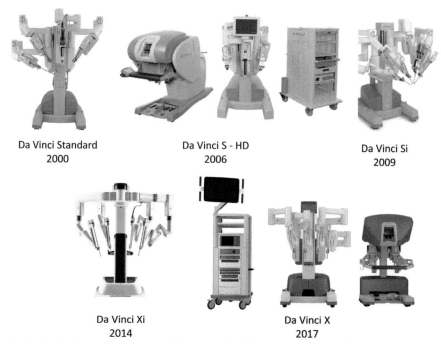

Da Vinci Standard
2000

Da Vinci S - HD
2006

Da Vinci Si
2009

Da Vinci Xi
2014

Da Vinci X
2017

**Fig. 1.** Da Vinci surgical systems. (*Courtesy of* Intuitive Surgical, Inc. Sunnydale, CA; with permission.)

From a procedure-specific standpoint, robotic hysterectomy (RH) in the United States increased from 0.5% of all hysterectomies in 2007 to 9.5% in 2010. More interestingly, in the 3 years following the first robotic procedure at hospitals where RH was performed, RH accounted for 22.4% of all hysterectomies.[3] This trend appears to hold true in countries around the world. In Korea, the number of robotic gynecologic procedures increased from 18 to 3860 in the first 13 years (2006–2019). The rate of yearly increase has been greater in the past 5 years with a 40% increase in robotic

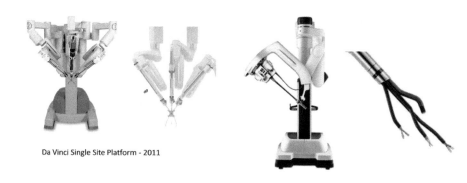

Da Vinci Single Site Platform - 2011

Da Vinci SP - 2018

**Fig. 2.** Da Vinci SP surgical systems. (*Courtesy of* Intuitive Surgical, Inc. Sunnydale, CA; with permission.)

procedures in 2019.[4] In Australia, robotic gynecologic surgery showed much more modest growth from 10 procedures in 2007 to 844 in 2016.[5]

Overall, since 2015, robotic surgeries have increased by almost 20% each year. The largest increases have been seen in general surgery, whereas transoral robotic surgery in ENT has shown the slowest uptake (**Fig. 3**).[4,6] In 2019, there were approximately 1,229,000 surgical procedures performed worldwide across all surgical specialties using the various da Vinci platforms.[6]

## ROBOTIC SURGICAL PLATFORM TODAY

Since 2000, there have been 4 generations of multiport da Vinci Surgical Systems, each with various enhancements (see **Fig. 1**). The original model, known as the Standard, had 3 arms: 2 instrument arms and a camera arm. A fourth arm was added in 2003. With the da Vinci S, the patient cart became less bulky, and visualization improved with an upgrade to a 3-dimensional (3D) high-definition camera. The da Vinci Si model added Firefly near-infrared fluorescence imaging capabilities as well as a dual console for teaching. The da Vinci Xi model changed the patient cart by mounting the instrument arms on an overhead boom to allow for more ergonomic positioning and multiquadrant access and added laser instrument targeting as well as subsequent enhancements to its EndoWrist instruments and electrosurgical capabilities.[7]

The da Vinci single-incision technology has also evolved to include significant improvements over the years. In its first iteration, known as Single-Site surgery, surgeons use modifications to the da Vinci Si and Xi platforms.[8] A specialized single-site port is used in conjunction with curved cannulae and semirigid, curved instruments.[9] Although minimally invasive, this approach poses limitations because of a lack of triangulation and the inherent challenges of placing instruments mounted to 3 robotic arms through a single umbilical incision. As a result, the recently released da Vinci Single Port (SP) system was developed to address these limitations by introducing integration of 3 instruments operated by a single robotic arm and a single cannula (see **Fig. 2**).

## THE INEVITABILITY OF COMPETITION

Inherent to technological evolution in the marketplace is the advent of newer robotic surgical platforms. As they seek to compete with the established da Vinci Surgical

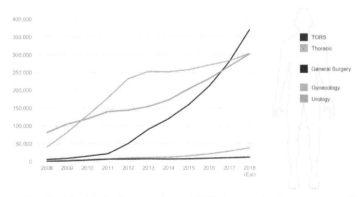

**Fig. 3.** Growth in Da Vinci Robotic procedures. TORS, transoral robotic surgery. (*From* Intuitive Surgical Inc. Annual Report 2018. Annu Rep. Published online 2018:122. https://www.annualreports.com/Company/intuitive-surgical-inc; with permission.)

Systems, several important areas are being targeted with new innovations: surgeon ergonomics, visualization, incorporation of haptic feedback, and reduction of the overall footprint, which includes making the robotic platform itself more compact as well as decreasing the size and number of incisions.[10,11] Some of these advancements will be discussed in further detail. Additional ventures aiming to combine virtual reality and artificial intelligence technologies to robotic surgery are also under development.

New and developing platforms on the near horizon with the potential for use in gynecologic surgery have been included in **Table 1**. The list is not exhaustive, with more competitors continuing to enter the arena with ventures, such as the Hugo system (Medtronic, Minneapolis, MN, USA) by Medtronic, announced in late 2019,[12] and the Ottava system (Johnson & Johnson, New Brunswick, NJ, USA), announced by Johnson and Johnson in late 2020.[13]

The Senhance Surgical System (Asensus Surgical, Durham, NC, USA) by TransEnterix received FDA approval in October 2017 and is currently the only other FDA-approved alternative to the da Vinci Surgical Systems in the United States. Thus far, single-center studies have shown safety and feasibility in general surgery, gynecology, and urology procedures with both 5-mm and 3-mm robotic instruments.[14,15] In addition to smaller instruments and trocar sizes, the Senhance system differs from the da Vinci platform in multiple ways that will be further detailed in later discussion.

In Europe, The Versius Surgical Robotic System (CMR Surgical, Cambridge, UK) by CMR Surgical and the Avatera (avateramedical GmbH, Jena, Germany) by avateramedical GmbH have both obtained CE Mark. All other platforms listed in **Table 1** have yet to obtain CE Mark and/or FDA approval. The Revo (meerecompany, Seoul, Korea) by meerecompany obtained clinical approval in 2017 but specific to its use only in Korea.

### Ergonomics and the Surgeon Console

One undeniable benefit of robotic surgery is its superior ergonomics when compared with conventional laparoscopy (**Fig. 4**). The physical demands of performing surgery are real and gaining more attention.[16] Poor ergonomics and increased and repetitive strain cause chronic pain and disability for many surgeons.[17,18] Surgeons are increasingly recognizing the benefit of robotic surgical platforms in reducing the cumulative wear their bodies experience as they tackle more complex pathologic conditions on patients with increasing body mass indexes (BMIs) (**Fig. 5**). Although surgeons performing minimally invasive surgery generally report less overall pain with use of the da Vinci Surgical System over traditional laparoscopy, studies continue to show areas of musculoskeletal strain with robotics as well. Ergonomic studies have demonstrated that surgeons continue to place a significant amount of strain on their bodies when performing robotic surgery because of poor ergonomics while seated at the robotic console for long periods of time.[19,20] Interestingly, 1 survey of gynecologic oncologists reported worse pain with robotic surgery than with laparoscopic surgery.[21]

When pain is reported with robotic surgery, it generally focuses on finger, neck, and back strain.[19,22–24] These areas of increased strain make sense when one considers the position the surgeon must take to sit at the da Vinci surgeon console. This positioning involves leaning forward into the eyepiece to achieve 3D visualization and reach the hand controls (**Fig. 6**). The hand controls use finger loops to mimic a pincer grip.

As with any surgical system, the lack of intentional optimization of the system's ergonomics to the user with resultant poor posture will lead to musculoskeletal strain and discomfort over time. These problems have the potential to become magnified if robotic surgery is preferentially used for larger and more complex pathologic

**Table 1**
Robotic surgical platforms on the market and in development

| | 3D Vision Technology | Surgeon Console Design | Ergonomy | Instruments | Patient Interface | Trocar Sizes (mm) | Haptic Feedback |
|---|---|---|---|---|---|---|---|
| *Multiport Platforms* | | | | | | | |
| Da Vinci Si, X, Xi Intuitive Surgical (Sunnyvale, CA, USA) FDA approved | Stereoscopic | Closed | • Seated, leaning forward<br>• Armrests<br>• Finger loops<br>• Foot pedals | Wristed 10 uses | Single cart 4 arms | 8 & 12 | No |
| Avatera avateramedical GmbH (Jena, Germany) CE mark | Stereoscopic | Closed eyepiece | • Seated, leaning forward<br>• Integrated seat<br>• Armrests<br>• Finger loops<br>• Foot pedals | Wristed Single use | Single cart 4 arms | 5 | Yes |
| MiroSurge Medtronic | Flat panel autostereoscopic display without use of glasses | Open | • Seated upright<br>• Finger loops<br>• Armrests<br>• Finger loops<br>• Foot pedals | Wristed Multiple uses Can also use standard handheld instruments mapped to the tips of the robotic instruments | 3–5 arms individually mounted on OR table | Trocar sizes unknown | Yes No haptic feedback with handheld instruments, only robotic hand controllers |
| Revo-I Meerecompany (Seoul, South Korea) Korean Ministry for Food and Drug Safety Approval | Stereoscopic | Closed | • Seated, leaning forward<br>• Armrests<br>• Finger loops<br>• Foot pedals | Wristed 20 uses | Single cart 4 arms | 8 | Yes |

*(continued on next page)*

**Table 1**
*(continued)*

| | 3D Vision Technology | Surgeon Console Design | Ergonomy | Instruments | Patient Interface | Trocar Sizes (mm) | Haptic Feedback |
|---|---|---|---|---|---|---|---|
| Senhance TransEnterix (Morrisville, NC, USA) FDA approved | Flat panel display with 3D glasses | Open | • Seated upright<br>• Hand controllers like laparoscopic instruments<br>• One foot pedal<br>• Eye-tracking camera control<br>• Head movements to zoom in and out | Non-wristed Unlimited use | Individual carts 4 arms | 3 & 5 instruments 10 camera | Yes |
| Versius CMR Surgical (Cambridge, UK) CE mark | Flat panel display with 3D glasses | Open | • Seated upright or standing<br>• Armrests<br>• Joystick controllers | Wristed No. of uses unknown | Individual carts 5 arms | 5 | Yes |
| *Single-Port Platforms* | | | | | | | |
| Da Vinci SP Intuitive Surgical (Sunnyvale, CA, USA) | Stereoscopic | Closed | • Seated, leaning forward<br>• Armrests<br>• Finger grips<br>• Foot pedals | Multijointed, wristed Articulating endoscope Multiple use | Single cart Single port/arm 1 camera 3 instruments | 25 | No |
| Enos (previously known as SPORT) Titan Medical Inc (Toronto, Canada) | Flat panel display with 3D glasses | Open | • Seated upright<br>• Armrests<br>• Hand and Finger grips | Flexible instruments and endoscope Single use instrument tips | Single cart Single port/arm 1 camera 2 instruments | 25 | Yes |

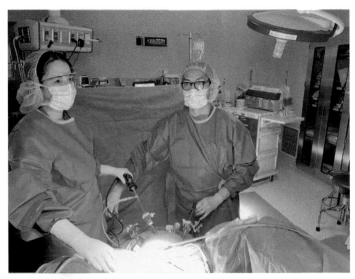

**Fig. 4.** Ergonomics with conventional laparoscopic surgery.

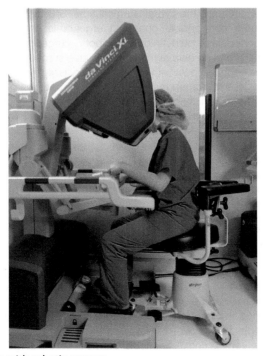

**Fig. 5.** Ergonomics with robotic surgery.

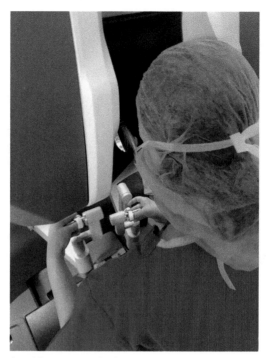

**Fig. 6.** Closed console with stereoscopic viewer.

conditions that may increase the overall surgical time. Studies have shown that when surgeons were more comfortable changing ergonomic settings to ensure ideal posture, they reported less pain following robotic surgery[25] and that ergonomic training and optimization can help significantly reduce surgeon pain.[18,22]

Notably, surgeon-reported pain with robotic surgery is significantly higher in women and in younger surgeons. Women make up a higher proportion of surgeons in gynecology than any other specialty in addition to making up a higher proportion of the younger cohort of gynecologic surgeons. They are also shorter and have smaller glove sizes on average than their male counterparts.[18,21] It has been shown that the da Vinci surgeon console is not ideal for shorter surgeons given the limited adjustments that can be made to bring foot pedals closer to the surgeon while remaining seated at the optimal distance for use of the hand controls and eyepiece.[25] An ergonomic study found that the robotic console allows for a comfortable posture only for individuals 64 to 73 inches in height.[26]

### Open versus closed consoles

As the limitations of the current surgeon console paradigm have been identified, new robotic platforms seek to make changes that target the designs that may lead to increased surgeon strain. In the da Vinci system, stereoscopic vision is achieved using a binocular endoscope where 2 cameras provide separate left and right images that are received by each respective eye using a binocular eyepiece. This requires a closed eyepiece that brings the images close to the surgeon's eyes so that they can be perceived as a single 3D image.

For example, the Versius and Senhance systems allow the surgeon to sit in an open console design versus being seated in a traditional closed console that forces the surgeon to lean forward to use a stereoscopic viewer. These systems use a flat panel display and 3D glasses to maintain 3D vision. The Senhance vision system also incorporates infrared eye tracking to control the camera and tracks forward and backward movement of the head to zoom in and out. The flat panel displays 2 interlaced images, and the lenses of the glasses are polarized at 90° to one another so that each eye only sees the image it is intended to see. Because of the way these images are interlaced with each other, the horizontal resolution of the image is halved but the vertical resolution is unchanged.[27] Polarized 3D flat screen images are subsequently less high fidelity and are not as bright. Open console designs may also allow taller surgeons to sit more comfortably without having to hunch forward to use closed stereoscopic eyepieces. In fact, the Versius system is unique in that it also gives the surgeon the option to stand at the surgeon console. Beyond potential ergonomic advantages, another benefit of an open console design may be improved interaction and communication with bedside assistants and other operating room (OR) staff since the surgeon's head is not immersed in the console. Although the Avatera system uses a stereoscopic viewer, it aims to improve communication by reducing overall noise and designing the console so that the surgeon's ears and mouth are not enclosed when the surgeon leans forward into the enclosed eyepiece.

*Hand controllers*
Some new robotic surgical platforms also use different configurations of hand and finger controls that reduce strain. The Versius Surgical Robotic System uses joysticks that integrate functions for clutching arms, arm switching, endoscope control, and diathermy all within the hand controller instead of separate foot pedals as in the case of the da Vinci and the Revo-I systems. By doing so, the ergonomic challenges experienced by shorter surgeons unable to reach foot pedals comfortably are addressed.

On the other hand, the Senhance system uses controls that mimic traditional laparoscopic instruments because the use of familiar controls was shown to decrease training time for surgeons already performing traditional laparoscopy.[11] However, as with traditional laparoscopy, the Senhance instruments are not wristed and lack the articulation and dexterity that many have come to expect with robotic surgery. As of yet, ergonomic studies have not been performed on these new robotic platforms, and comparisons to the da Vinci Surgical System cannot be made.

*Haptic Feedback*

A common complaint of robotic surgery is the lack of haptic feedback or tactile sensation whereby a surgeon can feel force, traction, tension, and slippage of tissues during surgery. Without haptic feedback, surgeons rely on visual cues to estimate, based on how the tissues appear to respond to manipulation, how much force has been applied. The widely used da Vinci Surgical Systems do not have haptic feedback.

The Senhance Surgical System has been shown to provide haptic feedback that is realistic, although possibly with a slight lag time in surgeon perception. This feature allows the surgeon to feel the force applied by instruments on the tissue through the hand controllers while also providing the capability to amplify the forces transmitted for increased sensitivity. Studies thus far have shown that the addition of haptic feedback does not adversely affect surgeon learning curve.[11,15,28,29] All other robotic systems mentioned here report the inclusion of haptic feedback into their respective platforms; however, information on their performance is not yet available.

*Decreasing the Robotic Surgical Footprint*

*Smaller robots*

As a growing number of companies enter the marketplace, many seek to decrease the overall size of robotic surgical systems in order to allow for easier use in smaller ORs. Reorganizing ORs or building new operating facilities to fit large patient carts and surgeon consoles can be expensive and difficult. Having a dual console in the OR for trainees is even more limiting. Modifications to the current paradigm thus far have included modular patient carts where each robotic arm is brought to the operating table on its own cart, thereby allowing surgeons to set up and use only the arms they need. The Senhance Surgical System, although modular, is still quite large. The Versius Surgical Robotic System is significantly smaller and more portable.

*Smaller instruments*

Smaller instruments allow for smaller trocars and less patient trauma. The Senhance Surgical System reports the smallest instruments thus far at diameters of 3 mm and 5 mm. However, the camera requires a 10-mm trocar. All other systems described thus far report instrument diameters in the range of 5 mm to 8 mm.

*Single-port robotic surgery*

The da Vinci SP has a single robotic arm through which 3 robotic instruments and a camera are placed through one 25-mm cannula. The instruments are wristed and elbowed, and the camera is also wristed for improved triangulation.[30,31] The SP platform was released in 2018 (see **Fig. 2**) and requires its own unique patient cart, surgeon console, and vision cart. The SP platform is only FDA approved for use in robotic urology and otolaryngology procedures. Single-institution studies of gynecologic procedures have shown feasibility and safety.[32,33] The surgeon console is similar to the other da Vinci platforms with instruments that can be swapped between hands by pressing a button on the instrument navigator interface.[34]

The Titan Medical Enos (Titan Medical, Toronto, Canada), formally known as the SPORT system, is a single-port platform that takes up a smaller OR footprint with a smaller and more mobile surgeon console than the da Vinci SP. Also, in contrast to the da Vinci SP, it has an open surgeon console and only 2 robotic instruments. The instruments are multiarticulated and are introduced through a camera insertion tube (CIT) that has a separate 2-dimensional (2D) wide-angle camera for use in addition to the 3D high-definition multiarticulating camera. The CIT with 2D camera can be used in the same way that an initial diagnostic laparoscopy might be used before robotic surgery to ensure feasibility of the procedure before placement of the 3D camera or instruments.[35,36]

*The Cost Debate*

It has often been argued that robotic surgery is more costly than laparoscopic surgery without justifiably significant improvements in outcomes.[3,37,38] Although an in-depth discussion of the financial implications of incorporating robotics into surgery is beyond the scope of this article, a comment must be made regarding the process by which early conclusions have been drawn. As an example, previous randomized controlled trials comparing RH to traditional laparoscopic hysterectomy (LH) were often performed at institutions where surgeons were highly skilled in LH but had very limited experience with RH, thereby completely ignoring learning curves.[39] Hence, it came as no surprise what the conclusions would ultimately be.

More recent studies limited to high-volume robotic surgeons have demonstrated shorter operative times, lower estimated blood loss, shorter length of hospital stay, and fewer postoperative complications with RH when compared with LH, even in the presence of worse adhesive disease, higher patient BMI, and larger uteri.[40–42] In a recent single-center analysis of high-volume, subspecialty trained gynecologic surgeons performing LH and RH, there were statistically significant differences in both mean direct cost and mean operating times for uteri larger than 250 g with even greater reductions in operating times and costs when RH was performed on uteri larger than 750 g. Most of the difference in cost was attributed to decreased operating time. However, the investigators also note that at this institution, effort has been made to reduce direct costs associated with robotic surgery where possible by using only the minimum necessary operative robotic arms and instruments and increasing awareness of cost among surgeons and OR staff.[40] Although further research is necessary, these findings are encouraging and highlight how complicated cost analyses can be, especially when attempting to conduct randomized controlled trials in surgery where multiple variables affecting the outcomes must be taken into consideration. Increasing surgeon experience, advancing technologies, and more competition in the marketplace have the potential to improve patient outcomes and reduce costs further. These discussions also argue for increased scrutiny regarding utilization of robotic surgical systems and the granting of hospital privileges to surgeons.

As more competitors enter the marketplace, production costs per surgical system will need to decrease along with the associated costs per procedure. Facilitating ease of setup, allowing surgeon customization specific to their needs, and providing extended-use instrumentation versus single use will also help drive down costs. **Table 1** lists instrumentation that can be used multiple times, although the number of uses before expiration is not known for all systems.

*Ensuring Safety: Credentialing and Robotic Surgery Privileges*

As an increasing number of innovative surgical platforms race to enter the market, ensuring the safety and efficacy of robotic surgery remains paramount, particularly regarding surgeon experience and the inevitable learning curves that come along with any new technology. The current and pending introduction of newer technologies makes current conversations around the credentialing and privileging process of surgeons even more important. Although guidelines exist to assist hospitals in developing robust privileging processes, current requirements for robotic surgery vary widely across the country and many are likely inadequate to ensure surgeon proficiency and patient safety. At many hospitals, surgeons meeting minimal requirements can gain global privileges for use of robotic surgical technology without limitation based on surgical procedures or ability to perform a procedure via conventional laparoscopy or laparotomy. Standardized and robust credentialing and privileging processes are recommended to ensure safe use of new technologies by properly trained surgeons.

According to The Joint Commission, the medical staff at each hospital holds ultimate responsibility for credentialing and granting hospital privileges to its employed physicians. However, it does not provide a specific structure, and existing processes are widely variable and often inadequate.[43–45] In 2013, a small FDA survey of surgeons performing robotic surgery with a da Vinci Surgical System revealed no standardization of credentialing processes across 11 individual institutions.[46] A 2020 review of 42 institutions from 24 states across the United States showed inconsistency for even basic requirements, such as whether a robotic training course was required, and, if so, what that training must entail.[43] The study pointed out significant inadequacies in existing credentialing policies to ensure surgeon proficiency and patient safety. For many years, specialty societies, including American Association of Gynecologic Laparoscopists (AAGL), the American Urological Association (AUA), the Society of

American Gastrointestinal and Endoscopic Surgeons, and the Minimally Invasive Robotic Association, have advocated for the development of and/or implemented guidelines to achieve a more uniform standard and ensure safe robotic surgery.[47–50] However, even among themselves, these specialty-specific guidelines are not uniform, and hospital uptake is unknown.

Recently, in 2020, a consensus conference of robotic surgery experts across multiple disciplines was convened to define uniform credentialing criteria for implementation across institutions. These experts agreed that there should be a separate credentialing process for robotic surgery and that a common credentialing pathway for basic robotic surgery across all specialties would be beneficial. Processes should be defined for initial credentialing for trainees, practicing surgeons, and maintenance of privileges.[51] Research has not identified a reliable minimum number of robotic cases needed to reach satisfactory performance. This is further complicated by the existing literature showing very large ranges of case minimums across surgical specialties that in turn also differ based on the surgical procedure in question. Therefore, proficiency should not be based solely on the number of cases performed.[50–52]

There was widespread agreement among consensus participants that before seeking robotic surgery privileges, surgeons recently graduating from residency or fellowship should be board certified or board eligible in their specialty (or appropriate equivalent) and those in practice or moving from a different institution should have documentation of an appropriate volume of cases with satisfactory outcomes. Regarding requirements for cognitive and technical training for robotic surgery, specialty societies have tackled this in varying ways (**Box 1**).

The recent consensus conference on robotic surgery also recommended proficiency-based training that relies on objective metrics of performance. They specified that such training should be developed by independent surgical education organizations and should not be left to device manufacturers. Device-specific training, however, should be sponsored by respective device manufacturers.[51] Simulation should be integrated as a part of any training, credentialing, and privileging pathway. With the advent of numerous low- and high-fidelity as well as virtual reality simulation platforms, necessary skills should be attained via simulation before they are performed in the OR. The consensus conference agreed that credentialing for new procedures should incorporate simulation and reliance on proficiency-based curricula. Specifically, the Fundamentals of Robotic Surgery curriculum was proposed as a future credentialing requirement. They also recommended that simulation should be used for both assessment and training should performance concerns arise.

Once privileges are attained, experts and specialty societies also agree that a surgeon's initial robotic cases should be monitored with initial cases performed under the supervision of a qualified preceptor (someone able to participate in the case in a hands-on fashion). Whether this process occurs in residency, fellowship, or as practicing surgeons, trainees or novices should participate in cases as first assistant before taking on the role of primary surgeon while the preceptor assists. Once proficiency is attained, initial cases should be monitored by an independent proctor before the surgeon performs cases independently. Initial independently performed cases should undergo peer review. The consensus conference specified that the proctor should not be picked by industry.

Regarding maintenance of privileges, specialty societies agree that surgeon proficiency should undergo continuous monitoring with a combination of minimum case volume requirements and outcome measures. However, guidelines are not specific regarding which metrics or outcome measures should be included, leaving this up to individual institutions.[47–49] The consensus conference found strong agreement

**Box 1**
**Guidelines for cognitive and technical training**

Society of American Gastrointestinal and Endoscopic Surgeons (SAGES) and the Minimally Invasive Robotic Association (MIRA)
  A formal robotic surgery training course should be taught by instructors with appropriate clinical experience and include didactic instruction as well as hands-on experience using inanimate and/or animate models.
  • Hands-on experience should include nonclinical simulation of system setup, operation, and troubleshooting.
  • Initial skill training should include basic and advanced techniques for proficiency in intended procedure.
  • Procedure-specific modeling should include successful completion of the key components using an appropriate model for the expected procedures.
  • Use advanced simulation tools when available.

AAGL Advancing Minimally Invasive Gynecology Worldwide
  • Complete an approved computer-based online training module
  • Complete at least 2 hours of bedside training by qualified trainer: docking, bedside assisting, and troubleshooting
  • Complete at least 1 hour of hands-on training with the robotic surgical system using inanimate training aids
  • Demonstrate competency on robotic simulator by passing specified skills drills (strongly encouraged, not mandatory)
  • Participate in a live pig laboratory course (unless documented previous robotic training as a resident or fellow)

American Urological Association
  • Complete AUA's Fundamentals of Urologic Robotic Surgery module with a posttest score of at least 80% correct
  • Recommend completion of at least one of the Basic Procedures modules of the AUA's Urologic Robotic Surgery Online Course for relevant robotic procedure with a posttest score of at least 80% correct.
  • Recommend completion of Intuitive Surgical's Online System Training Module, review of the Patient Preparation and Operating Room Setup for Laparoscopic and Robotic Surgery Chapter in the AUA's "Urologic Robotic Surgery Curriculum," and review of material specific to the robot type the urologist will be using in clinical practice.
  • Hands-on experience using the surgical robotic system with instruction by an instructor. This may include the following:
    ○ System set up and docking
    ○ Skills training using inanimate models and/or training with virtual reality simulators
    ○ Animal laboratory experience when available
    ○ Familiarity with robotic setup and technique for either or both upper urinary tract and lower urinary tract procedures depending on which the surgeon performs
    ○ Training with electrosurgical devices and other instrumentation that are used during the performance of robotic surgery

*Data from* Refs.[50,53,54]

that maintenance of privilege requirements should include an established annual robotic case volume, complication rates, estimated blood loss, operative time, rates of conversion to open surgery, rates of return to the OR, readmission rates, and operative costs. The expert panel recommended that institutions should develop acceptable performance criteria for these outcomes and that an audit of a surgeon be triggered if performance criteria were not met. The expert panel also recommended that all surgeons should undergo random performance audits in order to review operative performance via video-recorded cases using objective metrics at predetermined intervals.[51]

## SUMMARY

Robotic surgery has become an important part of the minimally invasive surgical landscape and promises only to expand its reach across almost all surgical disciplines and impact a myriad of procedures. New companies entering the marketplace are seeking to optimize surgeon ergonomics, improve visualization, provide haptic feedback, and overall make the robotic surgical systems smaller, cheaper, and more versatile. The integration of technologies like augmented reality and artificial intelligence, although still in the early phases of development, has the potential to truly advance surgical precision and therapeutic capabilities. Nevertheless, as we continue to aspire and to achieve these ambitious goals, we must take care to ensure that patient safety and surgeon training remain at the center. New technology cannot replace surgical skill. As our tools and technologies evolve and progress, it becomes even more important to use safeguards to ensure that indicated procedures are done using the proper tools in the hands of appropriately trained and proficient surgeons. We have much to look forward to. With these and future technologies at our fingertips, along with the new responsibilities they bring, we can continue to push the envelope toward exciting possibilities and new frontiers in gynecologic surgery.

## IMPORTANT DEFINITIONS

Credentials: Documented evidence of licensure, education, training, experience, or other qualifications.[53,55]

Clinical Privileges: Authorization by a health care organization allowing a health care practitioner to provide a defined class of patient care services.

Co-Surgeon: One of 2 or more surgeons working together to perform a specific procedure. Each co-surgeon assumes primary responsibility for that portion of the patient care and operative procedure that falls within their area of expertise.

Privileging: The process whereby a specific scope and content of patient care services (ie, clinical privileges) are authorized for a health care practitioner by a health care organization based on evaluation of the individual's credentials and performance.

Preceptor: An expert surgeon who undertakes to impart his/her clinical knowledge and skills in a defined setting to a preceptee. The preceptor must be appropriately privileged, board certified, skilled, and experienced in the procedure or procedures and/or technique or techniques in question. In order to serve as a preceptor in a specific procedure or technique, the surgeon (preceptor) must be a recognized authority (eg, publications, presentations, extensive clinical experience) in the particular field of expertise.

Proctor: An expert robotic surgeon that functions as an observer and evaluator, does not directly participate in patient care, does not serve simultaneously as a preceptor, and receives no fees from the patient. In rare cases, a proctor may intervene during a procedure on an emergency basis and assume responsibility for patient care in order to preserve the welfare of the patient.

Robotic-assisted surgery, robot, and robotic surgery: Terminology commonly used to refer to an advanced form of computer-assisted laparoscopic surgery or computer-assisted telesurgery or telemanipulation. These and other variants are often used interchangeably.

## CLINICS CARE POINTS

- As new robotic surgical systems enter the marketplace, challenges will exist not only with skill acquisition but also as it pertains to proper credentialing and privileging.
- High-volume robotic surgeons have demonstrated fewer complications with robotic hysterectomy compared to conventional laparoscopy.
- Given the physical demands of performing surgery, robotic surgical platforms can provide ergonomic advantages over conventional laparoscopy.

## DISCLOSURE

E.S. Han: The author reports no conflicts of interest. A.P. Advincula: The author reports the following relationships: Abbvie: consultant; Baxter: consultant; ConMed: surgeon advisory board/consultant; Cooper Surgical: consultant and royalties; Eximis Surgical: consultant; Titan Medical: surgeon advisory board/consultant; Intuitive Surgical: consultant.

## REFERENCES

1. Advincula, Arnold P, Song A. The role of robotic surgery in gynecology. Curr Opin Obstet Gynecol 2007;19(4):331–6.
2. Intuitive Surgical Inc. Annual report 2018. In: Annu rep. 2018. p. 122. Available at: https://www.annualreports.com/Company/intuitive-surgical-inc.
3. Wright JD, Ananth CV, Lewin SN, et al. Robotically assisted vs laparoscopic hysterectomy among women with benign gynecologic disease. JAMA 2013;309(7): 689–98.
4. Lee S, Kim M-R, Seong SJ, et al. Trends in robotic surgery in Korean gynecology. Gynecol Robot Surg 2020;1(2):50–6.
5. Nicklin J. The future of robotic-assisted laparoscopic gynaecologic surgery in Australia – a time and a place for everything. Aust N Z J Obstet Gynaecol 2017;57(5):493–8.
6. Intuitive Surgical Inc. Annual report 2019. 2019. Available at: https://isrg.intuitive. com/static-files/31b5c428-1d95-4c01-9c85-a7293bac5e05. Accessed February 8, 2021.
7. Varghese A, Doglioli M, Fader AN. Updates and controversies of robotic-assisted surgery in gynecologic surgery. Clin Obstet Gynecol 2019;62(4):733–48.
8. Jayakumaran J, Wiercinski K, Buffington C, et al. Robotic laparoendoscopic single-site benign gynecologic surgery: a single-center experience. J Robot Surg 2018;12(3):447–54.
9. Scheib SA, Fader AN. Gynecologic robotic laparoendoscopic single-site surgery: prospective analysis of feasibility, safety, and technique. Am J Obstet Gynecol 2015;212(2):179.e1–8.
10. Khandalavala K, Shimon T, Flores L, et al. Emerging surgical robotic technology: a progression toward microbots. Ann Laparosc Endosc Surg 2020;5:1–8.
11. Longmore SK, Naik G, Gargiulo GD. Laparoscopic robotic surgery: current perspective and future directions. Robotics 2020;9(2):1–22.
12. Hale C. Medtronic takes its new surgery robot out for a spin with investor debut. Fierce Biotech. Available at: https://www.fiercebiotech.com/medtech/first-look-medtronic-takes-its-new-surgery-robot-out-for-a-spin. Accessed February 1, 2021.

13. Sean W. Breaking: Johnson & Johnson finally unveils its new robot-assisted surgery system. MassDevice 2020;. https://www.massdevice.com/breaking-johnson-johnson-finally-unveils-its-new-robot-assisted-surgery-system/. Accessed January 24, 2021.

14. Montlouis-Calixte J, Ripamonti B, Barabino G, et al. Senhance 3-mm robot-assisted surgery: experience on first 14 patients in France. J Robot Surg 2019; 13(5):643–7.

15. Samalavicius NE, Janusonis V, Siaulys R, et al. Robotic surgery using Senhance® robotic platform: single center experience with first 100 cases. J Robot Surg 2020;14(2):371–6.

16. Park A, Lee G, Seagull FJ, et al. Patients benefit while surgeons suffer: an impending epidemic. J Am Coll Surg 2010;210(3):306–13.

17. Meltzer AJ, Susan Hallbeck M, Melissa M, et al. Measuring ergonomic risk in operating surgeons by using wearable technology. JAMA Surg 2020;155(5): 444–6.

18. Franasiak J, Ko EM, Kidd J, et al. Physical strain and urgent need for ergonomic training among gynecologic oncologists who perform minimally invasive surgery. Gynecol Oncol 2012;126(3):437–42.

19. Lawson EH, Curet MJ, Sanchez BR, et al. Postural ergonomics during robotic and laparoscopic gastric bypass surgery: a pilot project. J Robot Surg 2007;1:61–7.

20. Craven R, Franasiak J, Mosaly P, et al. Ergonomic deficits in robotic gynecologic oncology surgery: a need for intervention. J Minim Invasive Gynecol 2013;20(5): 648–55.

21. McDonald ME, Ramirez PT, Munsell MF, et al. Physician pain and discomfort during minimally invasive gynecologic cancer surgery. Gynecol Oncol 2014;134(2): 243–7.

22. Hokenstad ED, Hallbeck MS, Lowndes BR, et al. Ergonomic robotic console configuration in gynecologic surgery: an interventional study. J Minim Invasive Gynecol 2020. https://doi.org/10.1016/j.jmig.2020.07.017.

23. Wee IJY, Kuo LJ, Ngu JCY. A systematic review of the true benefit of robotic surgery: ergonomics. Int J Med Robot Comput Assist Surg 2020;16(4):e2113.

24. Catanzarite T, Tan-Kim J, Menefee SA. Ergonomics in gynecologic surgery. Curr Opin Obstet Gynecol 2018;30(6):432–40.

25. Lee MR, Lee GI. Does a robotic surgery approach offer optimal ergonomics to gynecologic surgeons?: a comprehensive ergonomics survey study in gynecologic robotic surgery. J Gynecol Oncol 2017;28(5):70.

26. Lux MM, Marshall M, Erturk E, et al. Ergonomic evaluation and guidelines for use of the daVinci robot system. J Endourol 2010;24(3):371–5.

27. Schwab K, Smith R, Brown V, et al. Evolution of stereoscopic imaging in surgery and recent advances. World J Gastrointest Endosc 2017;9(8):368–77.

28. Gueli Alletti S, Rossitto C, Cianci S, et al. The Senhance™ surgical robotic system ("Senhance") for total hysterectomy in obese patients: a pilot study. J Robot Surg 2018;12(2):229–34.

29. Hutchins AR, Manson RJ, Lerebours R, et al. Objective assessment of the early stages of the learning curve for the senhance surgical robotic system. J Surg Educ 2019;76(1):201–14.

30. Barrera K, Wang D, Sugiyama G. Robotic assisted single site surgery: a decade of innovation. Ann Laparosc Endosc Surg 2020;5:4.

31. Esther SH. Tech update: single port robot-assisted laparoscopic gynecologic surgery. AAGL NewsScope 2020;34(2). Available at: https://newsscope.aagl.org/volume-34-issue-2/tech-update-robotic-surgery/.

32. Misal M, Magtibay PM, Yi J. Robotic less and reduced-port hysterectomy using the da Vinci SP surgical system: a single-institution case series. J Minim Invasive Gynecol 2021;28(5):1095–100.

33. Shin HJ, Yoo HK, Lee JH, et al. Robotic single-port surgery using the da Vinci SP® surgical system for benign gynecologic disease: a preliminary report. Taiwan J Obstet Gynecol 2020;59(2):243–7.

34. Intuitive Systems - da Vinci SP. Available at: https://www.intuitive.com/en-us/products-and-services/da-vinci/systems/sp. Accessed January 18, 2021.

35. Seeliger B, Diana M, Ruurda JP, et al. Enabling single-site laparoscopy: the SPORT platform. Surg Endosc 2019;33(11):3696–703.

36. Discover Enos Technology. Available at: https://titanmedicalinc.com/technology/. Accessed January 18, 2021.

37. Khorgami Z, Li WT, Jackson TN, et al. The cost of robotics: an analysis of the added costs of robotic-assisted versus laparoscopic surgery using the National Inpatient Sample. Surg Endosc 2019;33(7):2217–21.

38. Wright KN, Jonsdottir GM, Jorgensen S, et al. Costs and outcomes of abdominal, vaginal, laparoscopic and robotic hysterectomies. J Soc Laparoendosc Surg 2012;16(4):519–24.

39. Paraiso MFR, Ridgeway B, Park AJ, et al. A randomized trial comparing conventional and robotically assisted total laparoscopic hysterectomy. Am J Obstet Gynecol 2013;208(5):368.e1–7.

40. Moawad GN, Abi Khalil ED, Tyan P, et al. Comparison of cost and operative outcomes of robotic hysterectomy compared to laparoscopic hysterectomy across different uterine weights. J Robot Surg 2017;11(4):433–9.

41. Klebanoff JS, Tyan P, Nishikawa M, et al. Cost variance across obesity class for women undergoing laparoscopic hysterectomy by high-volume gynecologic surgeons. J Robot Surg 2020;14(6):903–7.

42. Lim PC, Crane JT, English EJ, et al. Multicenter analysis comparing robotic, open, laparoscopic, and vaginal hysterectomies performed by high-volume surgeons for benign indications. Int J Gynecol Obstet 2016;133(3):359–64.

43. Huffman EM, Rosen SA, Levy JS, et al. Are current credentialing requirements for robotic surgery adequate to ensure surgeon proficiency? Surg Endosc 2020. https://doi.org/10.1007/s00464-020-07608-2.

44. Siddique M, Shah N, Park A, et al. Core privileging and credentialing: hospitals' approach to gynecologic surgery. J Minimally Invasive Gynecol 2016;23:1088–106.e1.

45. Sheetz KH, Dimick JB. Is it time for safeguards in the adoption of robotic surgery? HHS Public Access. JAMA 2019;321:1971–2.

46. FDA Center for Devices and Radiological Health. Final report: da Vinci surgical system 2013. Available at: https://www.fda.gov/media/87485/download.

47. Advancing A, Invasive M, Worldwide G. Guidelines for privileging for robotic-assisted gynecologic laparoscopy. J Minim Invasive Gynecol 2014;21(2):157–67.

48. American Urological Association. Robotic surgery (urologic) standard operating procedure (SOP). 2018. Available at: https://www.auanet.org/guidelines/robotic-surgery-(urologic)-sop. Accessed January 23, 2021.

49. Herron DM, Marohn M, Advincula A, et al. A consensus document on robotic surgery. Surg Endosc Other Interv Tech 2008;22(2):313–25.

50. Stefanidis D, Fanelli RD, Price R, et al. SAGES guidelines for the introduction of new technology and techniques. Surg Endosc 2014;28(8):2257–71.

51. Stefanidis D, Huffman EM, Collins JW, et al. Expert consensus recommendations for robotic surgery credentialing. Ann Surg 2020. https://doi.org/10.1097/sla. 0000000000004531.

52. Pernar LIM, Robertson FC, Tavakkoli A, et al. An appraisal of the learning curve in robotic general surgery. Surg Endosc 2017;31(11):4583–96.

53. AAGL. Guidelines for privileging for robotic-assisted gynecologic laparoscopy. J Minim Invasive Gynecol 2014;21(2):157–67.

54. American Urological Association. Robotic surgery (urologic) standard operating procedure (SOP). 2018. Available at: https://www.auanet.org/guidelines/robotic-surgery-(urologic)-sop. Accessed January 23, 2021.

55. Society of American Gastrointestinal Endoscopic Surgeons. The definitions document: a reference for use of SAGES guidelines 2009. Available at: https://www.sages.org/publications/guidelines/definitions-document-reference-for- use-of-sages-guidelines/.

# Professionally Responsible Counseling About Fetal Analysis

Frank A. Chervenak, MD, Laurence B. McCullough, PhD*

## KEYWORDS

- Ethical principle of beneficence • Ethical principle of respect for patient autonomy
- Fetal diagnosis • Fetal analysis • Fetal risk assessment • Maternal-fetal intervention
- Professional ethics • Professionalism

## KEY POINTS

- The pregnant patient is the ultimate decision maker about the performance of fetal analysis and the application of its results to her judgment about the disposition of her pregnancy.
- All pregnant women should be offered both noninvasive and invasive fetal analysis.
- When a pregnant patient refuses fetal analysis, the informed refusal process should be followed and documented in the patient's record.
- Shared decision making (offering but not recommending clinical management) should guide counseling about accepted maternal-fetal interventions.
- Shared decision making (offering but not recommending clinical management) should guide counseling about investigative maternal-fetal interventions.

## INTRODUCTION: ONCE AND FUTURE FETAL DIAGNOSIS

During the previous century, fetal diagnosis developed to classify normal and abnormal conditions of the fetuses. The results of fetal diagnosis served mainly to provide information that a pregnant patient could then use, with the counseling of her obstetrician, to make decisions about the disposition of her pregnancy.[1,2] These decisions were binomial: to end the pregnancy in induced abortion before viability or to continue pregnancy to term and plan for intrapartum and neonatal clinical management.[3,4] The most commonly chosen course of clinical management was induced abortion, suggesting a strong link between fetal diagnosis and termination of pregnancy.

Department of Obstetrics and Gynecology, Zucker School of Medicine at Hofstra/Northwell and Lenox Hill Hospital, 100 East 77th Street, New York, NY 10075, USA
* Corresponding author.
E-mail address: Laurence.McCullough@bcm.edu

Obstet Gynecol Clin N Am 48 (2021) 777–785
https://doi.org/10.1016/j.ogc.2021.06.005
0889-8545/21/© 2021 Elsevier Inc. All rights reserved.

obgyn.theclinics.com

In the past 2 decades, the scope of identification of the fetus's clinical condition has been expanded to include both diagnosis and risk assessment.[5] In addition, the scope of maternal-fetal intervention for fetal benefit has expanded beyond treatment of Rh immune disorder to include medical and surgical management of many conditions.

In this article, we use the phrase "fetal analysis" to refer to imaging and laboratory analysis, including genetic and genome analysis, to assess the anatomy and physiology of the fetus.[6] The results include risk assessment and diagnosis. These results are used by the obstetrician to identify maternal-fetal interventions with an evidence base of clinical benefit for the pregnant woman and, increasingly, the fetus and newborn. The pregnant woman's options are no longer binomial because they include further fetal analysis after risk assessment; further fetal diagnosis; induced abortion before viability; selective termination in utero of an affected fetus in multiple pregnancies; accepted maternal-fetal intervention; and experimental maternal-fetal intervention in the forms of either single-case innovation or multi-case approved clinical trials. We use "maternal-fetal" to underscore that medical and surgical interventions for fetal benefit must be done via the pregnant woman's body.[6,7]

Once, not long ago, professionally responsible counseling about fetal diagnosis was simple and well-understood: unbiased presentation of results and counseling about the 2 options described previously. Now professionally responsible counseling is about fetal analysis: unbiased presentation of results and counseling about the options described previously. This article draws on key concepts of professional ethics in obstetrics and gynecology to provide ethically justified, practical guidance to counseling pregnant women about fetal analysis. We begin with an overview of professional ethics in obstetrics and gynecology. We then deploy clinically relevant key concepts in professional ethics in obstetrics and gynecology to address when to offer and recommend fetal analysis and supporting pregnant woman to make informed and voluntary decisions about the clinical management of their pregnancies based on these results.

## PROFESSIONAL ETHICS IN OBSTETRICS AND GYNECOLOGY
### Origins in Eighteenth Century British Medical Ethics

Professional ethics in obstetrics is a subset of professional ethics in medicine, the invention of 2 British physician-ethicists in the late eighteenth century: John Gregory (1724–1773) of Scotland and Thomas Percival (1740–1804) of England.[6,8] Both responded to the long history of self-interested, entrepreneurial practice of medicine. Gregory, for example, starts his book on medical ethics with a sustained critique of physicians "of interest," that is, physicians who were motivated by self-interest. Percival criticizes what he calls "party interest" or the shared self-interests, for example, of physicians in competition with surgeons in the new, charitable hospitals in the United Kingdom, the Royal Infirmaries. By the mid-eighteenth century in Britain, medical practice was idiosyncratic, with almost as many concepts of disease and treatments as there were physicians. Pregnant women often paid the price, with their health and lives, and the lives of newborns. Gregory and Percival called for a powerful corrective to idiosyncratic practice: science-based practice. They appealed to the philosophy of medicine of Francis Bacon (1565–1626), who insisted that medicine be based on what Bacon called "experience," the results of observational and experimental clinical science. Science-based medicine also became an antidote to self-interested medicine.

Gregory and Percival wedded Bacon's philosophy of medicine to the moral philosophy of David Hume (1711–1776) to invent the ethical concept of medicine as a profession. This concept called for physicians to make 3 commitments: to becoming and remaining scientifically and clinically competent; to using their competence primarily for the good of the patient and to keeping individual self-interest systematically secondary; and to using their competence primarily for the good of the patient and to keeping party or group self-interest systematically secondary.[6] Making these 3 commitments transforms the sick individual into a patient, a human being who has been presented to a physician and there exist forms of clinical management that, in science-based clinical judgment, are reliably predicted to result in net clinical benefit. The ethical principles of beneficence and respect for autonomy translate these 3 commitments into clinical practice.

### Ethical Reasoning

Ethical reasoning aims to produce reliable judgments about what ought to be done, so that we do not have to rely on unsupported or mere opinion. The first step of ethical reasoning is to clearly formulate clinically relevant concepts. The second step is to identify the implications of these concept for clinical judgment and clinical management based on it.[6] Six ethical concepts are clinically relevant to professionally responsible counseling about fetal analysis: the ethical concept of being a patient; ethical principles; the ethical principle of beneficence in professional ethics in obstetrics; medically reasonable clinical management; the ethical principle of respect for patient autonomy in professional ethics in obstetrics; and the ethical concept of the fetus as a patient. See **Box 1**.

## SUPPORTING PREGNANT WOMEN'S DECISION MAKING ABOUT FETAL ANALYSIS AND ITS RESULTS
### Confidentiality

The patient should be assured that the existence of her early pregnancy and her decision about its disposition are completely confidential. Some patients may want to have her partner or others involved in the counseling process. The obstetrician should explain that they should maintain confidentiality just as the obstetrician will. This means that they are free to discuss what occurs only with the patient's explicit permission.[6]

### Clarifying the Patient's Role in Decision Making

The ethics of informed decision making in all clinical specialties is based on the ethical principle of respect for patient autonomy. This means that the patient is the ultimate decision maker. In this crucial role, her decision making should be voluntary, that is, free of controlling influences that might be asserted by others. These matters should be explained to the patient as the context for encouraging to involve her partner or others, if she so decides. When the patient brings her partner or another person to the counseling sessions, the obstetrician should explain that the patient is the ultimate decision maker and that the goal of the counseling process is to support the patient to make her own decisions.[6]

The pregnant patient's decision-making role applies when she is an adolescent. Applicable state law varies about the effect of pregnancy on removal of the status of being a minor. Some states hold that pregnancy emancipates, others do not, and still others are vague. States in the latter 2 categories may nonetheless stipulate that the patient is the decision maker for all clinical matters related to pregnancy, which can be interpreted broadly. Most parents, with the obstetrician's

---

**Box 1**
**Clinically relevant ethical concepts in professional ethics in obstetrics and gynecology**

*The Ethical Concept of the Being a Patient.* A living human being becomes a patient when he or she is presented to a physician and there exist forms of clinical management that are reliably predicted to benefit that human being clinically.

*Ethical Principles.* Ethical principles are action guides that generate ethical obligations, behavior that should occur because it is required. Absolute ethical obligations admit of no exception: the prescribed behavior should always occur. *Prima facie* ethical obligations do admit of justified exceptions: the prescribed behavior should occur unless ethical reasoning shows that another obligation should take precedence. Absolute ethical obligations are very difficult to justify. Almost all ethical obligations, therefore, are *prima facie*.[9]

*Ethical Principle of Beneficence in Obstetrics.* Percival was probably the first in the global history of medical ethics to use "beneficence." In obstetrics physicians have an ethical obligation to provide clinical management that is reliably predicted to result in net clinical benefit for the pregnant and fetal patients. Inasmuch as the reliability of this prediction is a function of evidence, the strength of beneficence-based ethical obligations varies directly with the evidence base for predicted outcomes.

*Medically Reasonable.* Clinical management that is supported in beneficence-based clinical judgment is known as medically reasonable.

*Ethical Principle of Respect for Patient Autonomy in Professional Ethics in Obstetrics.* Gregory expressed this ethical principle in nascent form when he called for physicians to acknowledge the right of patients to speak when their life or health is at stake. Physicians should listen and assess the patient's judgment on the basis of evidence for or against it. The ethical principle of respect for patient autonomy creates the *prima facie* ethical obligation to empower the female patient to make informed and voluntary decisions about the management of her clinical condition by providing her with information about the medically reasonable alternatives for its clinical management and the benefits and risks of each medically reasonable alternative.

*The Ethical Concept of the Fetus as a Patient.* The concept of the fetus as a patient is in the mainstream of the obstetrics literature, having appeared in journal articles and major textbooks for more than 4 decades. The acceptance of this concept is illustrated in the current edition of *Williams Obstetrics*, which includes a section with 8 chapters, "The Fetal Patient." The fetus becomes a patient when it is presented to an obstetrician or other health care professional and there exists forms of clinical management that are reliably predicted to benefit the fetus clinically. Before viability (approximately 24 weeks in high-income countries), the fetus becomes a patient solely as a function of the pregnant woman's voluntary decision to confer moral status on her fetus(es). After viability, the fetus becomes a patient when a pregnant woman is presented for clinical management. When the fetus is a patient, the obstetrician has 3 ethical obligations, *all of which must always be taken into account*: beneficence-based and autonomy-based *prime facie* ethical obligations to the pregnant woman and beneficence-based *prima facie* ethical obligations to the fetus.

Used with permission from McCullough LB, Coverdale JH, Chervenak FA. *Professional Ethics in Obstetrics and Gynecology.*

---

encouragement, will be supportive of their daughter's decisions and the patient will usually accept this support and benefit from it. Should parents attempt to usurp the patient's decision-making role, the obstetrician should make clear that the patient is the ultimate decision maker and protect her from undue influences that could undermine the voluntariness of her decisions.

Some states do not permit minor women to authorize termination of pregnancy without parental approval. Typically, these provide for a judicial bypass in which process the patient can petition the court to make her own decisions. Obstetricians should consult their organizational policy and their organizational legal counsel for guidance in this matter.

## Offering Fetal Analysis

To support autonomous decision making about the disposition of her pregnancy, every pregnant patient should be offered fetal analysis. This is an autonomy-based, not beneficence-based ethical justification. The obstetrician should explain the options in 3 clinical categories based on how the pregnant woman would experience them and their results.[5,6]

The first form of fetal analysis is noninvasive analysis of circulating fetal cells in maternal blood, obtained by standard blood draw. The second is ultrasound imaging, which is also noninvasive and usually performed in the first trimester. Second-trimester ultrasound should also be offered because it is more sensitive in detecting some fetal anomalies and its results can be used to make a decision of pregnancy before legal limits on induced abortion apply. By contrast, the third and fourth are invasive, to obtain early in pregnancy chorion villi from the placenta and later in pregnancy to obtain amniotic fluid that contains fetal cells. These need to be performed to allow time for results to be returned before legal limits on induced abortion apply.

The obstetrician should explain the kinds of results each form of fetal analysis produces. The most common result of analysis of fetal cells in maternal blood will be risk assessment, that is, a calculation of the risk of a fetal anomaly. To determine a diagnosis requires follow-up invasive fetal analysis, using either chorion villus sampling or amniocentesis. The obstetrician should explain that accepting this first form of noninvasive of fetal analysis does not commit the woman to accepting follow-up invasive analysis. She should be informed that circulating fetal cell analysis is the most sensitive screening test for Down syndrome or trisomy 21.

The results of ultrasound analysis include both risk assessment and diagnosis. In the first trimester, ultrasound is used to make a risk assessment for trisomy 21 and diagnoses such as anencephaly. In the second trimester, the examination is more thorough with a higher diagnostic yield. The results of both forms of invasive fetal analysis are diagnostic. With genomic and chromosome analysis, the diagnostic yield increases.

In response to the offer of fetal analysis, pregnant women should be expected to respond along one of the following decision-making pathways.[5,6,10] Some women will accept noninvasive fetal analysis for risk assessment, either by maternal blood sampling and/or ultrasound. The patient's informed decision should be implemented. Some women will prefer to obtain only diagnostic information, from 1 or more of ultrasound, chorion villus sampling, or amniocentesis. The patient's informed decision should be implemented.

Some women will refuse fetal analysis altogether. The obstetrician should fulfill the strict legal and ethical requirement of informed refusal by informing the patient that she is forgoing the opportunity to learn risk-assessment and diagnostic information about her fetus and will therefore be making subsequent decisions about the management of her pregnancy without this information. Specifically, she should be informed that she may not learn that her fetus is among the 2% to 3% with fetal anomalies that occur in pregnancies. She should also be informed that her refusal can be withdrawn later. This should be placed in the context of information about legal restrictions on access to termination of pregnancy under applicable law. This disclosure should be documented in the patient's record.

## COUNSELING ABOUT RESULTS OF FETAL ANALYSIS: THE ESSENTIAL ROLE OF SHARED DECISION MAKING

Counseling about the fetus's condition and how that information should be presented has been, and continues to be, governed by the ethical standard of nondirective counseling. This long-accepted ethical standard is based on the ethical principle of respect for patient autonomy, buttressed by the reality that the obstetrician is not competent to decide whether a woman should remain pregnant when her fetus is affected by an anomaly or disorder. To empower the pregnant woman to exercise her autonomy, the obstetrician should present results in an unbiased fashion and refrain from making any recommendation, even if directly asked. The patient should be supported to draw on her own values and beliefs to assess the results of fetal analysis and her alternatives. This is a classic example of the application of shared decision making, understood as unbiased presentation of results and refraining from making any recommendation.[6,9] This approach should be followed by all results, including the confirmed diagnosis of a lethal fetal anomaly.

## HOW TO COUNSEL ABOUT ACCEPTED MATERNAL-FETAL INTERVENTION

Some forms of maternal-fetal intervention are well established and life-saving for the fetus, such as intrauterine transfusion for severe anemia due to Rh isoimmunization. When a woman does not elect to terminate such a pregnancy, she has conferred the moral status of being a patient on her fetus. There is a beneficence-based ethical obligation to the fetal patient to recommend intervention that is life-saving. When making a recommendation, counseling becomes directive and shared decision making is not the ethically justified approach.

Spina bifida is a diagnosis for which there are now 2 medically reasonable alternatives, based on the results of the MOMS trial.[11] Antenatal surgery and neonatal surgery are not life-saving but are designed to prevent disability. They have differing benefit/risk profiles for pregnant, fetal, and neonatal patients. Antenatal surgery is more risky for the pregnant patient, whereas neonatal surgery is less effective in preventing shunting for hydrocephalus and thus preventing disability. When there are 2 medically reasonable alternatives, the ethical principle of respect for patient autonomy creates the *prima facie* ethical obligation to offer both to the pregnant woman who has elected to continue her pregnancy, explain their clinical benefits and risks of both, and support the patient to understand and evaluate each alternative. The difference in benefit/risk profiles means that neither should be recommended; there is no current, decisive evidence of superior clinical benefit for pregnant, fetal, and neonatal patients of one over the other. Directive counseling is therefore not ethically permitted; shared decision making should be the approach taken by the obstetrician.

## HOW TO COUNSEL ABOUT INNOVATION AND RESEARCH ON MATERNAL-FETAL INTERVENTION

Maternal-fetal intervention has made rapid technological advances in the past 2 decades. These interventions are at various stages of development. Given the rarity of conditions for which maternal-intervention is technically feasible, these interventions should be classified as experimental. By this we mean that the current evidence base does not support a reliable prediction of net clinical benefit for pregnant, fetal, and neonatal patients. An experiment can be performed on a single patient with the intent to benefit that patient. This is the definition of clinical innovation.[6] An experiment can also be performed with the intent to create generalizable knowledge. This is the definition of clinical research.[6]

Because innovation and clinical research on maternal-fetal interventions are experimental, there is no beneficence-based ethical obligation to the fetal patient to offer them, because there is no beneficence-based ethical obligation to any patient to offer, much less recommend, an experiment. However, there is an autonomy-based ethical obligation to explain to a pregnant woman whose fetus might qualify for innovation or clinical research that these opportunities exist. This information empowers the pregnant woman to consider this approach and request referral to fetal centers offering innovation and clinical research.

Pregnant women interested in innovation or clinical research should be informed that both are experiments, as defined previously. This means that she has no beneficence-based ethical obligation to her fetus to accept innovation or enroll in a clinical trial and also violates no ethical obligation to her fetus should she decide to decline innovation of enrollment in a clinical trial.

The obstetrician should explain that federal law required that only clinical research that has prospective review and approval by what is known as an Institutional Review Board is permitted.[12] In 2008, the Society of University Surgeons proposed that all planned surgical innovation should be undertaken only with similar prospective review and approval by a committee created for this purpose.[13] The authors have proposed that fetal centers should create Perinatal Innovation Review Committees to fulfill this function as a way of assuring pregnant women that innovation offered to them has been peer-reviewed for its scientific, clinical, and ethical justification.[6] This minimal disclosure will prepare the pregnant woman for the decision-making process she will experience if she contacts a fetal center.[14] The North American Fetal Therapy Network (NAFTNet) maintains a Web site with information about member centers.[15]

## ANTICIPATING THE FUTURE OF RESEARCH ON MATERNAL-FETAL INTERVENTION

Obstetricians should be prepared for 2 aspects of the future of research on maternal-fetal interventions. The MOMS trial may become a paradigm in which future clinical research on other maternal-fetal interventions results in adding a medically reasonable antenatal intervention to medically reasonable neonatal intervention. This may occur, for example, should current or future clinical trials produce results of clinical benefit for antenatal maternal-fetal surgery. The benefit/risk profile of antenatal and neonatal intervention will differ, because of the risk to pregnant women of antenatal intervention and the risk to the newborn of postponing surgery to the postnatal period. In this paradigm, counseling should be nondirective, as explained previously about the MOMS trial.

Genome science has led to the creation of techniques to alter the anatomy of the genome.[16] Research has been conducted on sickle-cell disease in adults with initial success and proof of principle.[17] The technological capacity to alter the genome of in vitro embryos and in utero fetuses will continue to develop. It will be crucial, as this development continues, that enthusiasm (the belief in clinical benefit in the absence of evidence for clinical benefit) be prevented. The language used will be very important, because some word choices promote enthusiasm. Consider, for example, "gene editing." This is an analogy to editing a written text in which letters and words are changed by an editor, only those letters and words are changed, the changes are permanent once the editing process has been completed. The function of these permanent changes itself does not change. None of this is true for altering the genome. There are "off-target" effects of technologies, such as clustered regularly

---

**Box 2**
**Criteria for innovation and early-phase clinical research of maternal-fetal interventions for fetal benefit**

1. The proposed fetal intervention is reliably expected on the basis of previous animal studies either to be life-saving or to prevent serious and irreversible disease, injury, or disability for the fetal patient.

2. Among possible alternative designs, the intervention is designed in such a way as to involve the least risk of mortality and morbidity to the fetal patient.

3. On the basis of animal studies and analysis of theoretic risks both for the current and future pregnancies, the mortality risk to the pregnant woman is reliably expected to be low and the risk of disease, injury, or disability to the pregnant woman is reliably expected to be low or manageable for current and future pregnancies.

Used with permission from McCullough LB, Coverdale JH, Chervenak FA. *Professional Ethics in Obstetrics and Gynecology.*

---

interspaced short palindromic repeats, known as CRISPR. The "letters" and "words" do not always go where they are intended to go. It is a standard dictum in the relationship between anatomy and physiology, unexpected changes in anatomy can result in unexpected changes in physiology, including unexpected pathophysiology. Finally, the changes to the genome may not be permanent.

The authors have proposed criteria to guide innovation and early-phase (safety and efficacy trials) research on maternal-fetal interventions[6,7] (**Box 2**). These are based on the ethical concept of the fetus as a patient. This ethical concept requires that the risk to the pregnant woman is minimized, as it is the to the fetal patient. In addition, in beneficence-based clinical judgment, given maternal risk, the priority should be on serious fetal conditions for investigation. The criteria are also in accord with US federal regulations for human subjects research.[12]

## SUMMARY

The clinical assessment of the fetus, or fetal analysis, now includes an impressive array of analytical tools to perform risk assessments and determine diagnoses. In addition, investigative maternal-fetal medical and surgical intervention continues to expand. Professional ethics in obstetrics and gynecology is an essential component of counseling pregnant patients about fetal analysis and referral for investigative maternal-fetal interventions. This article has drawn on the conceptual tools of professional ethics in obstetrics and gynecology (see **Box 1**) to provide practical, ethically justified guidance for the decision-making process with pregnant patients.

## CLINICS CARE POINTS

- Shared decision (nondirective counseling) should guide all aspects of counseling pregnant patients about fetal analysis.

- The obstetrician should involve others in the counseling process with the patient's permission, which may be implicit.

- The obstetrician should avoid enthusiasm (belief in clinical benefit in the absence of evidence) about investigative maternal-fetal interventions.

- The obstetrician should avoid his or her personal bias from influencing the counseling process.

## DISCLOSURE

The authors have nothing to disclose.

## REFERENCES

1. Screening for fetal chromosomal abnormalities: ACOG practice bulletin summary, number 226. Obstet Gynecol 2020;136:859–67.
2. American College of Obstetricians and Gynecologists' Committee on Practice Bulletins—Obstetrics, Committee on Genetics; Society for Maternal-Fetal Medicine. Screening for fetal chromosomal abnormalities: ACOG practice bulletin, number 226. Obstet Gynecol 2020;136:e48–69.
3. Chervenak FA, McCullough LB. An ethically justified practical approach to offering, recommending, performing, and referring for induced abortion and feticide. Am J Obstet Gynecol 2009;560:e1–6.
4. Chervenak FA, McCullough LB. Ethical dimensions of first-trimester fetal aneuploidy screening. Clin Obstet Gynecol 2014;57:226–31.
5. Nicolaides KH, Chervenak FA, McCullough LB, et al. Evidence-based obstetric ethics and informed decision-making by pregnant women about invasive diagnosis after first-trimester assessment of risk for trisomy 21. Am J Obstet Gynecol 2005;193:322–6.
6. McCullough LB, Coverdale JH, Chervenak FA. Professional ethics in obstetrics and gynecology. Cambridge and New York: Cambridge University Press; 2020.
7. Chervenak FA, McCullough LB. An ethically justified framework for clinical investigation to benefit pregnant and fetal patients. Am J Bioeth 2011;1139–49.
8. Chervenak FA, McCullough LB, Brent RL. The professional responsibility model of obstetrical ethics: avoiding the perils of clashing rights. Am J Obstet Gynecol 2011;205:315.e1–5.
9. Chervenak FA, McCullough LB. The unlimited-rights model of obstetric ethics threatens professionalism. BJOG 2017;124:1144–7.
10. Chervenak FA, McCullough LB, Sharma G, et al. Enhancing patient autonomy with risk assessment and invasive diagnosis: an ethical solution to a clinical challenge. Am J Obstet Gynecol 2008;199:19.e1–4.
11. Scott Adzick N, Thom EA, Spong CY, et al, for the MOMS Investigators. A randomized trial of prenatal versus postnatal repair of myelomeningocele. N Engl J Med 2011;364:993–1004.
12. U.S. Department of Health and Human Services. Office for Human Research Protections. 45 CFR 46. Available at: 45-CFR-46.HHS.gov, Accessed January 29, 2021.
13. Biffl WL, Spain DA, Reitsma AM, et al, Society of University Surgeons Surgical Innovations Project Team. Responsible development and application of surgical innovations: a position statement of the Society of University Surgeons. J Am Coll Surg 2008;206:1204–9.
14. Moise KJ Jr, Johnson A, Tsao K. Certification process of fetal centers in texas and developing national guidelines. Obstet Gynecol 2020;135:141–7.
15. North American Fetal Therapy Network (NAFTNet). Available at: North American Fetal Therapy Network (NAFTNet) NAFTNet, Accessed January 29, 2021.
16. Collins FS, Doudna JA, Lander ES, et al. Human molecular genetics and genomics - important advances and exciting possibilities. N Engl J Med 2021;384:1–4.
17. Frangoul H, Altshuler D, Cappellini MD, et al. CRISPR-Cas9 gene editing for sickle cell disease and β-Thalassemia. N Engl J Med 2021;384:252–60.

# Social Media Superpowers in Obstetrics and Gynecology

Meadow Maze Good, DO, FACOG[a,b,*], Staci Tanouye, MD, FACOG[c,d]

## KEYWORDS

• Physicians • Social media • Advocacy • Education • Empowerment

## KEY POINTS

• Social media is a ubiquitous form of communication and should leveraged wisely by the healthcare community for public health information.
• Patients are relying on social media for support, community, and health information.
• Health care providers have a duty to provide public health education by actively contributing accurate and reliable sources of health information to social media platforms.
• Health care providers must be aware of the pitfalls of social media and observe institutional policies on professionalism and social media.
• When used correctly, social media can be a powerful tool for communication, connection, and professional networking.

Social media has become a ubiquitous form of communication in our society and is an integral part of how we interact and engage. The term "social media" was first used in 2004 and added to the Merriam-Webster dictionary in 2011, defined as "forms of electronic communication (such as Web site for social networking and microblogging) through which users create online communities to share information, ideas, personal messages, and other content (such as videos)".[1] Social media platforms are powerful tools that instantaneously connect local and international communities, allowing the rapid dissemination of news, education, and resources, including health information. An obstetrician-gynecologist (ob-gyn) is undisputedly a leader and hero, caring for others and sharing their wealth of knowledge and experience on a daily basis. Offices full of women and their families wait patiently for their allotted time for a face-to-face interaction and advice. While they wait, they surf the internet and search social media

Disclosure: No commercial or financial conflicts of interest. No funding sources.
[a] ABOG Board Certified in Obstetrics & Gynecology and Female Pelvic Medicine & Reconstructive Surgery, 1404 Khul Avenue, 2nd Floor, MP 95, Orlando, FL 32806, USA; [b] Winnie Palmer Hospital for Women and Babies, OrlandoHealth, Orlando, FL, USA; [c] ABOG Board Certified in Obstetrics & Gynecology; [d] Women's Care of Florida, 5369 Bentpine Cove Road, Jacksonville, FL 32224, USA
* Corresponding author.
E-mail address: meadowgood@gmail.com

Obstet Gynecol Clin N Am 48 (2021) 787–800
https://doi.org/10.1016/j.ogc.2021.07.007
0889-8545/21/© 2021 Elsevier Inc. All rights reserved.

obgyn.theclinics.com

apps for available information on the health topic that consumes them. With over 4 billion people worldwide using social media each month (an average of approximately 2.5 hours per day), the opportunity for physicians to build their brands as health experts and use these platforms to connect with the public is imperative to population health, advocacy, and fulfilling the oath to care for people.[2] As depicted in **Fig. 1**, social media should be viewed as the superpower that it is; the remarkable ability to lift a finger and instantly connect the public with medical professionals sharing their expertise and therefore increasing medical comprehension and informed decision-making. Putting medical knowledge in a relatable way on the internet and social media sites for anyone to use empowers patients and strengthens the doctor-patient relationship by increasing communication and trust. The increased power of communication with social media allows the medical community to help guide patients before and long after they have seen their physician and medical team in the examination room. Additionally, social media platforms offer the obstetrician-gynecologist an opportunity to connect with peers, find support on a personal and professional level, and create safe places for professional networking.

Social media use is now widely prevalent among physicians for both personal and professional purposes. It is estimated up to 90% of physicians are on social media. Similarly, 90.4% of Millennials, 77.5% of Generation X, and 48.2% of Baby Boomers are using social media.[3,4] Originally, the use of social media among the physician community was in a personal capacity, sharing personal life events, experiences, and thoughts. Recently, physicians are using the platforms in a professional capacity to share health education with the public, create professional and patient communities, network, demonstrate examples of life in medicine, and market themselves and their practices. We are in a time when creating public trust in science, vaccination, and public health advisements is critical. Thus, advancing physicians' knowledge of using social media effectively is important to continued leadership in their communities. Please refer to **Box 1** for the recognized definitions of digital and social media technologies per the American College of Obstetricians and Gynecologists Committee Opinion, 791.

If physicians are not leading the dissemination of health information on social media, others less knowledgeable will fill the void and promote inaccurate and harmful information. *The charge is on the health care community, specifically obstetrician-gynecologists, to use social media as a powerful tool to connect and educate the public with accurate health information and resources.*

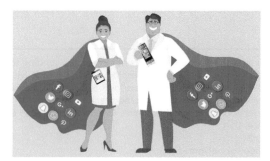

**Fig. 1.** Social media is a formidable tool and superpower that physicians should use for optimal communication, connection, and professional networking. (*Designed by artbesuro; Image #23234221 at VectorStock.com*)

---

**Box 1**
**Definitions**

*Digital media*—forms of electronic media where data are stored in a digital (as opposed to analog) format. The term can refer to the technical aspect of storage and transmission of the information (eg, hard disk drives or computer networking) or to the end product, such as digital video, augmented reality, digital signage, digital audio, or digital art. Web sites or web pages and social media often are considered a subset of digital media.[a]

*Social media*—forms of electronic communication, such as Web sites for social networking and microblogging, through which users create online communities to share information, ideas, personal messages, and other content.[b]

*Mobile media*—forms of electronic media accessed through a mobile device, such as a smartphone or tablet. This term encompasses social media sites that users access through a device's Internet browser or web-based applications (apps), as well as mobile device digital communication, such as text-messaging or short message service (commonly known as SMS).[c]

*Personal online profile*—an online profile, commonly created in the context of a social media outlet, that personally identifies an individual and represents that individual in online communication. A personal profile often is directed toward family and friends, although in some cases, it may be viewed by any online audience. Common examples of social media outlets that feature personal profiles include Facebook, Twitter, YouTube, and Spotify.

*Professional online profile*—an online profile, used in social media outlets, that pertains to a business, organization, or professional identity and that represents the entity primarily for professional purposes. Compared with a personal profile, a professional profile generally is directed to a public audience, such as an organization's membership, business clients or desired customers, or a physicians' group of patients. Such profiles may be used, for example, in social media sites, such as Facebook and Twitter, as well as professionally oriented sites such as LinkedIn and Doximity.

[a] University of Guelph. Digital media. Guelph (ON): university of guelph; 2006. Available at: http://www.uoguelph.ca/tss/pdfs/TBDigMedia.pdf. Retrieved August 27, 2014.
[b] http://www.merriam-webster.com/dictionary/social%20media. Retrieved August 27, 2014.
[c] Kaplan AM. If you love something, let it go mobile: mobile marketing and mobile social media 4x4. Bus Horiz 2012;55:129–39.

---

Social media use for health-related reasons has increased exponentially. A systematic review found social media use by patients effects the health care professional and patient relationship by leading to more equal communication between the patient and health care professional, increased switching of doctors, harmonious relationships, and suboptimal interaction between the patient and health care professional.[5] Health information on the internet and social media platforms spreads rapidly, often going completely unvetted. Health consumers are constantly searching for information, guidance, and resources, highlighting the need for professionals with vast education and experience to spread accurate information in this space and lead the public to informed decision-making. In a review of Instagram posts on miscarriage, a significant overarching theme to these posts was finding a source of support and community on a topic that is not discussed openly.[6] As social media continues to grow, so does the diversity and reach of the health topics covered. In one study on fertility education on Instagram, Peyser and colleagues examined the different types of posts on the topic of fertility.[7] Using top key terms, they found over 3 million posts on the topic of infertility. Of all the posts, 67% were posted by patients and only 10% by physicians, 4.5% by allied health professionals, and 1% by professional societies. From this, 60% of posts were related to patient experiences while only 8% were deemed educational.[7] This highlights the educational opportunity that physicians have to positively contribute to social media platforms. While Instagram is excellent for building new communities based on common interests, much of this interest is focused on personal experience. This community can be an excellent source of support; however, it is inevitable that health questions will arise. When they do, the question remains, "Who is providing the answers?" This is the space that medical professionals need to fill to ensure accurate health information is disseminated especially during the most vulnerable of times and sensitive subjects.

Women's health information is particularly vulnerable to misinformation, and obstetrician-gynecologist physicians tend to be less active in a professional capacity on social media than other medical specialties.[8] In order for our patients to find accurate health information and connect with their providers, the physicians need to be present in the spaces where patients are sharing their knowledge and experiences in a relatable, yet professional, way. The relatable experiences a physician would share with patients in an examination room to encourage good health practices (the patient who had a fetal demise, why we should not eat our placentas, or the reasons why you gave your daughter the Human Papillomavirus (HPV)) can be shared on social media platforms to impact millions of lives with one click. Engaging topics that trend from popular ob-gyn physicians on social media range from "female vulvovaginal anatomy" and "what not to put in your vagina" to "postpartum recovery" and "pregnancy loss." Our society benefits from our ob-gyn leaders engaging in social media, destigmatizing the discussions around women's health and creating open dialog around abortion, sex, and other sensitive female health issues.

Social media platforms are the optimal way to advocate on behalf of women and women's health inside and outside the examination room; engagement improves the lives of our patients and their families through spreading accurate health information and advocating for health policies that positively impact our communities. Additionally, physicians are leaders in our communities, which now includes the social media community, and have the ability to educate, support, and unite those affected by a particular illness or condition.

## SOCIAL MEDIA PLATFORMS

The various social media apps and platforms offer unique abilities to both physicians and professional organizations to rapidly disseminate crucial information to the public and to professionals during times of health care crisis (Coronairus Disease 2019 [COVID-19]). Each platform provides the opportunity to connect with communities worldwide to foster collegiality with peers or the possibility to offer life-changing and lifesaving medical information. You truly can unleash your superpower knowledge with cost- and time-effective social media platforms. As highlighted in **Table 1**, each social media platform has different strengths, weaknesses, and audiences.

## BUILD YOUR BRAND

A physician's social media accounts should lead to a cohesive message of who she/ he is as a person and professional and what your life's work is about. It should present a clear and consistent voice. Building a social media presence will also build your professional brand and what you are known for. Your brand will illustrate your education,

**Table 1**
**Comparative characteristics of different social media platforms**

| Social Media Platforms | | |
|---|---|---|
| Platform | Monthly Active Users | Highlights |
| Facebook | 2.7 billion | + Business page & ad features, personable, community<br>- Organic growth is harder, limited reach |
| YouTube | 2 billion | + Long video, built for educators, monetization potential<br>- Time-consuming, requires equipment, slower growth |
| Instagram | 1.1 billion | + Visually based, story-telling, community connections<br>- Time-consuming, not link-friendly, need lots of content |
| TikTok | 1 billion | + Short video, quick growth, large reach, young audience<br>- Time-consuming, creativity, quickly changes with trends |
| Pinterest | 440 million | + Good for SEO, discovery, higher conversion rates<br>- Narrow audience, time-consuming, increased spam |
| Twitter | 350 million | + Quick to use, fast-paced, professional connection<br>- Organic growth is difficult. 280 character limit |
| LinkedIn | 260 million | + Focuses on professional and career-related networking<br>- Smaller reach, not meant for patient connection |

abilities, and talents; highlight your achievements; reflect your strengths; create connection with your patients; and help network with your peers. Your brand can include a logo to represent you for advertising and promotion purposes. Having a positive message online can help combat any negative reviews one may receive. Claiming your online ratings (when possible) and responding to reviewer comments in a nonspecific way is helpful for showing you care and combats any negativity. Being ready for the inevitable public scrutiny is beneficial; regularly searching your name using search engines is recommended to know what is being said about you, your practice, and your brand. A relationship with a social media marketing company may be beneficial if you do not have the time or interest in "googling" yourself often or creating your own content. As social media evolves, physicians must be ready to adapt and create content needed to confirm their online credibility and presence. Once you get going and see the positive results, you will want to create more and engage more. Once you put yourself out there, do not be surprised if your next patient says, "I loved reading your tweets last week about women's health. Thank you!"

## FACEBOOK

Facebook is arguably the beginning of social media. While it certainly was not the first platform to exist, it is the one that set the stage for the entire digital social media industry. To put it in medical terminology, Facebook is the gold standard of social media. Launched on February 4, 2004, it started as a social platform to connect college students and initially required a ".edu" email address. Within 10 months, it reached 1 million users, and the rest is history. It rapidly outgrew its academic roots and was opened to everyone on September 26, 2006. With the development of community connection through Facebook Photos, Mobile, News feed, Groups, Messenger, and the concept of the "Like" button, Facebook solidified itself as the foundation of social media. By the end of 2012, it reached more than 1 billion active users and also acquired Instagram.[9]

Facebook is currently the largest social media platform in almost every way with over 2.7 billion monthly users.[2] Outranked by Google and YouTube, Facebook continues to be where many of our life-long patients are looking for and sharing information. As of January 2021, 54.7% of all Facebook users self-identified as female with the largest demographic being women of reproductive age, many of whom are here talking about their pregnancies, health care concerns, and health tips.[10] One of the largest strengths of Facebook is the ability to create public and private groups, which not only fosters community with people of common interests but also builds small business communities. With the increased popularity of "Groups", there is a Facebook group for almost every hobby, interest, or health care issue. Through member-created groups, the social media platform has created a safe place for patients with breast cancer and other serious medical illnesses to find information and support. Medical professionals have used the groups' function to build exclusive membership communities for their own personal businesses, coaching services, mentorship services, as well as professional clubs. It is also a powerful marketing tool with the average user clicking on 12 Facebook ads per month. If you and your practice do not have professional Facebook pages, do not delay and build one today.

Pro Tip: Create a business page and attach it to your personal page. If your primary business is your practice, make it practice oriented. If you have a personal brand or business, make your business page your personal brand page.

### YouTube

Are you tired of saying the same thing over and over and have considered recording yourself so you can share what you know with your patients? With over 2.0 billion monthly active users and over a billion hours of video viewed daily, YouTube offers the ability to showcase your talents and knowledge without being repetitive.[11] YouTube was founded in 2005 and was bought by Google in 2006. YouTube saw the value and rise of video very early on and quickly captured the video market. They were the first social media platform to create a partnership program with its most popular creators as way to support their creators not only creatively but also financially through various monetization opportunities. As video becomes more important to daily life, YouTube continues to evolve with the needs of their users.[11]

Medical professionals and institutions have used YouTube as a teaching tool extension. Educational, instructional, and even surgical videos on every health topic imaginable can be found on YouTube. Current medical creators provide a mix of traditional educational topics, updates on current medical events, fact-checking of popular culture trends, and even reactions to television medical dramas. Merging entertainment with medical accuracy has proven a popular niche in social media and continues to grow.

Pro Tip: Establish a regular posting schedule so your followers know when to expect your videos to be published. This creates a loyal and reliable follower base.

### INSTAGRAM

Unlike its desktop-based Facebook predecessor, Instagram is a visual story-telling platform optimized for mobile devices. Founded in 2010, it quickly proved the appeal of visual photo-sharing and became part of the Facebook family in 2012.[12] In fact, "instagramming" has earned its way into the dictionary as a verb.[13] While other social media platforms are built off of communities who know each other or are personally linked in some way, Instagram is unique by reaching wider communities of similar interests via something called the "Explore page." The Instagram Explore page is an endless page of curated posts and videos that you may not have otherwise seen. Scrolling through an explore page will provide a user with content chosen for them by an algorithm based on their previous actions and interests within the app. This allows an expanded exposure to other users with similar interests but may not otherwise be personally connected.

With over 1.1 billion active monthly users currently, Instagram is used by individuals, celebrities, artists, businesses both small and large, news organizations, educational institutions, and even medical professionals.[2] By focusing on photo-sharing with a caption character limit, visual content can be easily and quickly digested. About 60% of users will follow a new brand after seeing an appealing ad, and more than one-third have purchased something directly from an Instagram ad, making it a very effective marketing tool. The health industry has readily adapted to this format providing a mixture of personal health experiences with health education and healthy lifestyles promotion. Researchers have used Instagram and other visual platforms to study the impact on public health imagery from everything from disease states to vaccinations and mental health.[14] This platform is a valuable tool to reach the obstetric patient population who are busy researching their pregnancy needs and planning the arrival of their new baby. Sensitive and important ob-gyn health-related subjects are discussed on this platform including sexually transmitted diseases, breastfeeding, and pelvic floor disfunction. Instagram is a great space for ob-gyns to introduce themselves, their talents, personalities, and passions to their patients. Giving accurate health tips and education on Instagram can go a long way and be shared many times over. Engagement on this platform is based on how much you want to engage and are willing to give; the possibilities are limitless.

Pro Tip: Organic growth can be slow but is well worth the patience. Avoid the temptation to buy followers and likes. While it may sound like a quick path to a successful audience, it will do the opposite by effectively decreasing your engagement rate and pushing you further down in the algorithm so your content will be viewed even less by your actual followers.

## TikTok

TikTok is one of the newest social media platforms. It is a social media app that focuses on short-form videos on any topic one can imagine. TikTok is the product of the merging of two different Chinese companies, originally designed around music, dancing, and lip-syncing into the TikTok we know today. The most downloaded social media app today is a platform of 3- to 60-second videos on virtually any topic conceivable.[15] It is estimated to have nearly 1 billion monthly active users and was the most downloaded social media app in 2020, surpassing giant Facebook.[2,16,17]

The value for an ob-gyn using this platform is engagement with a younger population on health education topics and increasing health literacy. In the United States, 60% of TikTok users self-identify as female, and 80% are between the ages of 16 and 34 years, a key demographic for sexual and reproductive health education.[17] Teaching this demographic by meeting them where they are, and on their terms, engages them in a more relatable way. This encourages them to seek more reliable information that is both fun and medically accurate. In a time when science is in question and sexual health barely taught, physicians have the opportunity to showcase their personal or office staff's talent encouraging the public to seek medical attention and teach about important health topics.

Pro Tip: Tiktok's algorithm favors videos that are watched all the way through to completion as well as videos that are shareable. The best way to achieve this is to hook viewers within the first 2 to 3 seconds with a fun fact, question, or action to peak their interest and keep them watching. In order to ensure they finish watching your video, keep it short, to the point, and punchy.

## TWITTER

Tweeting your thoughts about a unique, once-in-a-lifetime surgical case or how you helped a senior get vaccinated may spark a conversation with another physician or even a patient. Twitter is the fastest, most interactive social media app with freely flowing conversations based on hashtags and followers. You can tweet the #MedTwitter community a clinical scenario to ask for out-of-the-box ideas or share a joke. There is room for sharing health information including #vaccine information and #advocacy views as legislation is being debated pertaining to women's health. The American College of Obstetricians has multiple Twitter handles including @acog and @acognews to reach its members, the community, and politicians. Many professional society meetings live tweet their annual meetings to engage their members and share news with the public. It is a great source of camaraderie and information. Twitter has the ability to bring the medical community together with patients and industry in a way that no other platform does. It will continue to grow as a place for physicians, especially ob-gyns, to find others with similar interests interested in education, innovation, and collaboration. Your Twitter feed is made of people you "follow"; your "followers" are those interested in your posts. The more you interact with others, the more you will build a following.

Pro Tip: Engage and connect with other medical professionals on #MedTwitter by not only tweeting thoughts and questions from your account but also by replying and conversing with others. Use relevant hashtags and tag accounts who may be interested in the topic of your tweet or answering your question. Follow accounts with similar interests and engage with others to build a following.

## PINTEREST

Pinterest is a social media Web site and app for sharing and categorizing images and interests, as a visual "bookmarking site." Pinterest categories include home design, art, crafts, cooking, fashion, travel, and, of course, many others including health topics. This platform is useful if you want to share with your audience health tips including recipes, exercise sites, specific products you recommend, or meaningful branding information. Pins are added to your board that can lead viewers to your Web site, blog, and other social media sites. Descriptions on the intentions of your board and pin will drive others looking for those topics to your site. Using relevant keywords will show your pins and board to your desired audience and help to build traffic on this and your other social media sites. When trying to describe your page, try to use one sentence summarizing what your page is about (you have up to 500 characters for your Pin description). For instance, "Looking for a credible source in women's health to guide you in maximizing your healthy lifestyle choices? Dr Good is an experienced obstetrician-gynecologist with a passion for low-carbohydrate cooking and outdoor activities for the entire family." An algorithm behind the scenes will use the words in your description to drive traffic to your board that will engage and share your pins and information.

Pro Tip: Share your favorite educational resources as a pin with an easy-to-understand description and keywords that describe you and your mission. The more specific your keywords are, the better for increasing meaningful traffic to your Pinterest board.

## BLOGS/WEB SITES

With so many social media options, why does anyone need a Web site with a blog? The Web site (possibly with a blog) is the opportunity to tie all your social media experiences together and broadcast your brand from one central location. Creating a Web site that reflects your passions as an ob-gyn and simultaneously reflect your interests on a personal level will embody your brand, integrating all your messaging from various platforms. It can be a place your patients come for educational information and a place for you to reflect on your life's purpose. Many ob-gyns who are successful on social media have a Web site that gives the viewer a complete picture of who the person is professionally and personally. You can make it as in-depth or superficial as you want. The Web site is your canvas to opening your life to the world. There are many different popular sites to create a Web site or blog (Wordpress, Blogger, Blogspot, Wix, Wordpress, and Squarespace). Using your full professional name is encouraged for easy identification by search engines, and creating something you enjoy looking at is the key to making it a fulfilling project.

Pro Tip: Use your Web site as a resource with links to all your social media handles. Create an email list to capture people who visit your blog or Web site and want to learn more or stay in touch. This is one of the few sources of followers that you own and can keep without relying on a separate social media company.

### Professional Networking

Many professional social media networking applications exist. LinkedIn is used by every professional industry including banking and real estate. The medical profession has quickly adapted to connecting via LinkedIn for career expansion or networking opportunities. Although it is not the main site for physician networking, it does continue to be a valuable source for developing relationships with hospital administration and busines opportunities. Doximity is a physician-only app, with a public profile and a private side that allows physicians to share research, successes, and communicate with encrypted messaging, inbound and outbound fax capabilities, phone dialer with a caller ID and phone number of your choosing, and a career center. Additionally, there are many ways to connect with physician peers on Facebook (including secret invite-only groups), Instagram, and Twitter.

Pro Tip: Connect with local colleagues and possible referral sources via Doximity. Establish a "Caller ID" so you can use your private cell phone labeled as an office phone number to call patients and fax pharmacies. Keep your LinkedIn profile up-to-date if you are in the job market or looking for career opportunities.

### Social Media Risks

Being engaged with and participating in social media platforms is not without risk. Performing complex pelvic surgery on a live woman is also not without risks. Social media allows another level of intimacy into the medical world, one that many have no idea exists. There may be people who do not agree with your practices or posts as an ob-gyn. However, the benefits of participating and voluntarily sharing on social media your knowledge and understanding of the field you have spent so much of your life studying and practicing far outweighs the risks. Flooding the platforms with science and accurate health information impedes the misinformation and allows the public to continue to see the physician as a leader both in the community and online. Physicians have been reprimanded by state medical boards for unprofessional behavior on social media platforms, usually by violating patient's privacy and/or confidentiality. Violations in the Health Information Portability and Accountability Act (HIPAA) by posting any patient identifiable health information may be accidental or unintentional, but is always avoidable. Complaining about patients or posting compromising photos of patients is never okay, and fortunately negative experiences with social media is the minority. Physician interaction with social media is an opportunity to engage, educate, and market themselves.

## PROFESSIONALISM

Physicians are health care heroes. Obstetrician-gynecologists care for women throughout their lives and through some of their most sensitive life experiences. Social media is a powerful tool that allows important health messages to be disseminated quickly; it is important to be mindful of your target audience and the purpose of your social media accounts. Being candid, relatable, and informative is important. Continuation of the professional values physicians hold themselves accountable for in the hospital setting is also recommended online. Be aware of your specific institution's social media policy to avoid professionalism issues. Many hospital systems are encouraging physicians and the other hospital staff to post about their work stories but avoid patient-identifying information. HIPAA violations should be avoided by speaking generally about a specific medical topic and not including any identifying information about a particular case. If you searched, many examples exist describing when a physician posted a compromising photo or complained about a patient with identifying information, and the patient/family member has complained to the news media and the state medical board. This simply should not ever be done. Social media has been around more than 15 years; the profession has learned from its mistakes and encourages sharing within the known boundaries that a physician should not cross when referring to medical care or patient-related care. Never be specific or share identifying information. Educate on the topic but leave people, places, and time out. A popular theme on social media is to portray "A Day in the Life of a Physician," by walking through a doctor's day step by step. While this is an important theme, it is also worth noting that these should be fictional representations of what a day in the life of a physician could look like and should never exactly mimic a specific day or case. When in doubt, leave it out.

Giving medical advice without knowing the person's full medical history or misrepresenting credentials are ways that a physician may be reported to the state medical board. When a physician creates a professional social media profile, naturally there are people who see it as a way to ask their own personal health questions and may even send direct messages asking about their own health concerns. Answering these types of questions should be avoided. In general, giving health tips and answering educational questions on social media is encouraged and supported by health organizations. Taking the time to share credible resources and educational sites will only improve public understanding of serious medical conditions and strengthen the trust in the medical community.

Additionally, refrain from posting illegal, intoxicated, or irrational behavior. Showing how to work hard and enjoying life is relatable, but posts may be interpreted in a way that was not intended and taken out of context. Sharing personal information and photos on social media has not only allowed medical professionals, including physicians, a window into their daily lives of caring for others but also shows how they are human and relatable. Showcasing sense of humor, struggles with ups and downs, health issues, and juggles of everyday life just like everyone else is accepted, encouraged, and may even help patients connect to their physicians in a way that builds a stronger foundation of trust. But be mindful that your actions may be magnified because of your position in your community as a health care hero. If you desire a robust social media presence, it is equally important to share your medical knowledge and your ability to connect with your patients on a personal level. Building a following on social media occurs when your content and personality are on display in a transparent and engaging way.

In 2020, a prominent medical journal issued an apology after a published article titled "Prevalence of unprofessional social media content among young vascular surgeons" sparked the #MedBikini movement where women physicians posted themselves in bikinis and holding alcoholic beverages. This backlash was to protest the statement that unprofessional photos included "provocative posing in bikinis/swimwear" and "holding/consuming alcohol." Many argued that the contents of the article targeted women and highlighted the problem of sexism in the medical field. This movement created important dialog in the medical community and public regarding sexism, professionalism, and social media content.[18]

On social media, physicians are promoting self-care to their colleagues as much as they are to their patients; this includes posts that are transparent regarding work-life balance, self-love, time-away, and struggles with infertility, weight, and health issues including mental illness. Social media has the power to touch a person's life and provide context and resources to positively impact decisions they may not have otherwise. Being professional includes being transparent with the many sacrifices you make to care for others. Showing your career achievements though hard work, dedication, and sacrifice can motivate and inspire others; also demonstrating how you strive to have a normal balanced life like the rest of the population is also welcomed. Be mindful of your superpower as showing continuous frustration or disrespect regarding your daily sacrifices may not be well received. Before you publish your thoughts on social media, THINK, is the content True, Helpful, Inspiring, Necessary, and Kind? It is important now as it ever has been to "pause before you post" to ensure when you click the send button, you will not have regrets. Most posts by physicians are encouraging and compassionate, highlighting the compassion of our field. It may be helpful to refer to a quick checklist (**Fig. 2**) before publishing a post on social media.

*Social Media Advocacy*

Social media is a powerful tool to advocate for our patient's best interests both inside and outside the clinical setting. One example of this tool used effectively is when Planned Parenthood, an organization known to most ob-gyns for its mission to provide preventative services to community members in need, took to the social media platforms to ask for help. In 2012, the Susan G. Komen's Race to the Cure organization announced that they were defunding the Planned Parenthood organization in a policy mismanagement. Planned Parenthood quickly went to social media platforms and announced that they were being attacked and needed support to provide the many preventative services they are known for including breast cancer screenings. Millions of Planned Parenthood supporters rallied on Facebook and Twitter. In 3 days, the Planned Parenthood organization raised 3 million dollars, and Susan G. Komen apologized and reversed their decision.[19] There are multiple simple ways to support women's health through advocacy on social media. Supporting specific hash tags including #InternationalWomensDay or #SheforShe or #HeForShe promotes equality and brings awareness of women's health and their important position in society. Most recently, physicians have united using #ThisisOurShot to show support in receiving the COVID-19 vaccine and encouraging the public trust science and receive

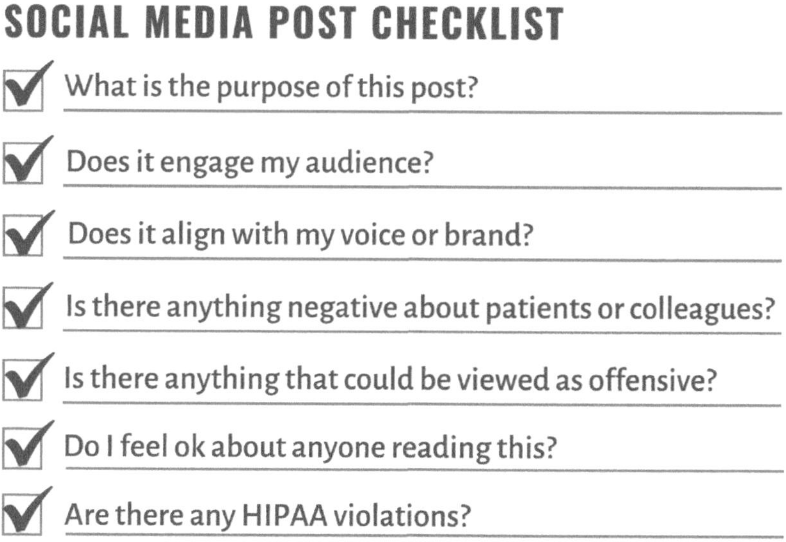

# SOCIAL MEDIA POST CHECKLIST

☑ What is the purpose of this post?

☑ Does it engage my audience?

☑ Does it align with my voice or brand?

☑ Is there anything negative about patients or colleagues?

☑ Is there anything that could be viewed as offensive?

☑ Do I feel ok about anyone reading this?

☑ Are there any HIPAA violations?

**Fig. 2.** A checklist to review before publishing a post on social media.

the vaccine when it is their turn. Social media is an effective tool to promote change and public empowerment.

Many health care organizations regularly use social media to advocate for better health care practices through sharing health information and using their voice to advocate for health policy. Both the American College of Obstetricians and Gynecologists and the American Board of Obstetrics and Gynecologists have social media accounts on the top platforms. Leveraging our patient relationships (and politicians' constituents) on their preferred platform of communication allows open dialog of topics that are up for debate including maternal and postpartum care, insurance coverage, maternal morbidity and mortality reviews, abortion, and preventative service access. Ob-gyns must continue to do what they do best: advocate for and take care of women. This includes influencing patients and their families by sharing important messages and political challenges on social media platforms. As they say in Washington DC, "If you are not at the table, you are on the menu."

### Future Superpower of Social media

The world without social media will never exist again. As telemedicine and social media use by physicians continues, the impact and reach will only positively affect women and their families if physicians choose to engage and be a part of the social media community. The superpower of social media should be harnessed and taught as a valuable tool in medical school and residency. Similar to the learning curve of any medical procedure, social media proficiency and expertise develops after education and repetitive use. As highlighted in the Key Points, social media is a mainstay of communication and should be leveraged as the superpower that it is to increase medical literacy and trust among our patients. As soon as this article is published, it will become outdated; social media is quickly changing, engaging, and becoming more interactive on multiple levels. The future of social media as it relates to health care is intriguing. As in-person meetings continue to decrease and the use of telemedicine flourishes, perhaps the future doctor office waiting room is a social media platform where patients interact and learn about their providers and various health topics. For physicians to direct the movement of public health information and policy, they must not just be involved but leading. Now is the time for physicians to create profiles, interact, and share knowledge. This interaction can positively build brands for the physician, clinic, and hospital system they are affiliated with.

## CLINICS CARE POINTS

- Social media is a powerful tool that can be utilized to advocate for our patient's best interests both inside and outside the exam room.

- Using social media as a physician comes with professional responsibility governed by institutional policies and the state medical board.

- Patients use social media to help them find a physician and credible health information to guide their decision making.

## REFERENCES

1. Professional Use of Digital and Social Media: ACOG Committee Opinion, Number 791. Obstet Gynecol 2019;134(4):e117–21.
2. Social Media Benchmark Report 2021. Influencer Marketing Hub. Available at: https://influencermarketinghub.com/ebooks/IMH_SOCIAL_BENCHMARK_REPORT_2021.pdf. Accessed August 23, 2021.
3. Surani Z, Hirani R, Elias A, et al. Social media usage among health care providers. BMC Res Notes 2017;10(1):654.
4. Bosslet GT, Torke AM, Hickman SE, et al. The patient-doctor relationship and on-line social networks: results of a national survey. J Gen Intern Med 2011;26(10):1168–74.
5. Kofinas JD, Varrey A, Sapra KJ, et al. Adjunctive social media for more effective contraceptive counseling: a randomized controlled trial. Obstet Gynecol 2014;123(4):763–70.
6. Mercier RJ, Senter K, Webster A, et al. Instagram Users' Experiences of Miscarriage. Obstet Gynecol 2020;135(1):166–73.
7. Peyser A, Goldstein L, Mullin C, et al. Fertility education: what's trending on Instagram. Fertil Res Pract 2021;7(1):3.
8. Yadav GS, Nagarkatti NR, Rohondia SO, et al. Academic tweeting in #ObGyn. Where do we stand? J Perinat Med 2019;47(8):867–70.
9. Facebook: Who We Are. Available at: https://about.fb.com/company-info/. Accessed August 23, 2021.
10. Tankovska H. Distribution of Facebook users in the United States as of January 2021, by gender. (2021, February 1). Available at: https://www.statista.com/statistics/266879/facebook-users-in-the-us-by-gender/. Accessed March 1, 2021.
11. YouTube by the numbers. (2021, February 1). Available at: https://blog.youtube/press. Accessed March 1, 2021.
12. Instagram: About us. Available at: https://www.instagram.com/about/us/. Accessed August .23, 2021.
13. "Instagram." Merriam-Webster.com Dictionary, Merriam-Webster. Available at: https://www.merriam-webster.com/dictionary/Instagram. Accessed August 23, 2021.

14. Fung, IC, Ahweyevu JO, Duke CH, et al. Public Health Implications of Image-Based Social Media: A Systematic Review of Instagram, Pinterest, Tumblr, and Flickr. Perm J2020;24:18.307.

15. What is TikTok? - The Fastest Growing Social Media App Uncovered. Available at: https://influencermarketinghub.com/what-is-tiktok/. February 1, 2021.

16. Kemp S. Digital 2021: Global Overview Report 2021. Available at: https://datareportal.com/reports/digital-2021-global-overview-report. February 1, 2021.

17. TikTok Statistics. Available at: https://wallaroomedia.com/blog/social-media/tiktok-statistics/#:~:text=Monthly%20Active%20Users%20%E2%80%93%20%20TikTok%20has,of%20now%20(January%202021. February 6, 2021.

18. Johnson LM, Ebrahimji. A medical journal apologized after an article prompted health professionals to post images of themselves in bikini.CNN. 2020. Available at: https://www.cnn.com/2020/07/25/cnn10/medbikini-backlash-and-apologies-trnd/index.html. August 23, 2021.

19. Komen Foundation restores funding for breast cancer screenings at Planned Parenthood Health Centers. Available at: https://www.plannedparenthood.org/about-us/newsroom/press-releases/komen-foundation-restores-funding-for-breast-cancer-screenings-at-planned-parenthood-health-centers. August 23. 2021.

# Infertility Treatment Now and in the Future

Kevin J. Doody, MD[a,b,*]

## KEYWORDS

• Artificial intelligence • Embryo culture systems • In vitro fertilization • IVF

## KEY POINTS

• Increased success in the treatment of infertility has been brought about by pharmaceutical development, new surgical techniques / instrumentation and improved assisted reproductive technology procedures.
• IVF has become the preferred treatment for many causes of infertility including sperm issues, egg / hormonal problems as well as anatomical abnormalities (endometriosis and tubal factors).
• Creation of artificial gametes through stem cell technology may soon allow application of assisted reproductive techniques in patients whose gametes have been depleted.

## INTRODUCTION

Understanding how fertility treatment has evolved to present day provides clues as to how treatments likely will continue to progress in the future. In many instances, improvements came through refinement and optimization of existing treatments. In other cases, technological breakthroughs allowed the development of entirely new treatments. This article puts the evolution of fertility treatments into a broad historical context. The likely continued refinement and optimization of current treatments are discussed with a focus on in vitro fertilization (IVF). Finally, recent disruptive technological breakthroughs in animal models are discussed.

## HISTORY

Human fertility has been regarded by many cultures as of utmost importance because it is essential for the survival and perpetuation of mankind. Fertility gods were ubiquitous in nearly all ancient human cultures and were used to help understand fertility and to cope with infertility through rituals and offerings.[1] The earliest change in the approach to dealing with infertility was seen in ancient Egypt. Unlike other civilizations, infertility was not considered divine punishment but rather an illness that merited diagnosis and treatment.[2] The Kahun papyrus is part of a group of medical texts originating

[a] CARE Fertility, 1701 Park Place Avenue, Bedford, TX, USA; [b] University of Texas Southwestern Medical Center, Harry Hines Boulevard, Dallas, TX, USA
* CARE Fertility, 1701 Park Place Avenue, Bedford, TX.
E-mail address: kevind@embryo.net

Obstet Gynecol Clin N Am 48 (2021) 801–812
https://doi.org/10.1016/j.ogc.2021.07.005
0889-8545/21/© 2021 Elsevier Inc. All rights reserved.

obgyn.theclinics.com

in Egypt approximately 4000 years ago; it discusses pregnancy, with prescriptions for conception that include incense, fresh oil, dates, and beer.[3]

The Renaissance marked a period of scientific and medical progress. *De Humani Corporis Fabrica* was published by *Vesalius* in 1543.[4] This anatomic atlas included cross-sections of the female genital organs. In 1672, de Graff wrote *De Mullerium Organis*, in which he described the ovary and follicular function. These publications marked the true beginning of the scientific study of reproduction.

The mechanism of the occurrence of pregnancy was not established until Antonie van Leeuwenhoek constructed the first simple microscopes. In 1677, van Leeuwenhoek made the first description of sperm and sperm motility. At the time, it was thought that fertilization occurred from vapors arising out of the seminal fluid.[5] He was the first to hypothesize that sperm actually penetrate the egg. This placed him in direct conflict with scientists who felt that the egg was the sole source of new life.

## BACKGROUND
### Artificial Insemination

van Leeuwenhoek's concept of fertilization ultimately led to attempts at pregnancy through the use of artificial insemination approximately 100 years later. It seems appropriate to consider artificial insemination the first practical, science-based infertility treatment. The first successful insemination was reported in a dog by the Italian physiologist Lazzaro Spallanzani in 1784.[6] John Hunter of London wrote the first report of artificial insemination in humans in 1790. He described a successful pregnancy through the collection of semen and subsequent injection via a syringe into the vagina in a case of infertility resulting from severe hypospadias.

In 1943, Alan Guttmacher of Johns Hopkins University published, "The Role of Artificial Insemination in the Treatment of Human Sterility."[7] Artificial insemination was becoming widely applied by that time. For many years, insemination with semen was indicated only in cases of retrograde ejaculation, vaginismus, hypospadias, and impotence. Insemination with semen from unrelated donors was employed in cases of male sterility. Although this treatment was found highly effective, perceived moral and legal issues hindered the widespread application of donor insemination for many years. During this time, techniques adopted in animals were applied to humans. Despite the demonstration of success in the horse, no human successes were documented with this technique.

In 1949, Polge and colleagues[8] introduced a simple method of preserving human sperm using glycerol as a cryoprotectant. Sherman used this technique to achieve a pregnancy in humans in 1953.[9] It was another 3 decades before this technique was translated more widely into the creation of commercial donor sperm banks. The delay was related to social, ethical, and moral concerns regarding donor insemination. Another source of delay was lower pregnancy rates using thawed sperm for cervical insemination. This changed with the realization that intrauterine insemination (IUI) of the thawed sperm restored "more normal" fertility. Ultimately, the safety from infectious disease enabled by sperm freezing and quarantine has made the use of fresh donor semen obsolete.

### Intrauterine insemination

Techniques of semen processing developed for the purpose of IVF advanced and widened the use of IUI with sperm from the male partner.[6] These "washing" procedures removed contraction-inducing prostaglandins while removing sperm with absent or reduced motility. The result of this type of sperm preparation was to broaden the indications for artificial insemination. IUI following semen processing first was reported to be successful for unexplained and mild male factor infertility in the mid-

1980s and this led to widespread adoption as a first-line treatment.[10] IUI with husband sperm remains one of the most applied fertility treatments worldwide despite some controversy remaining about its effectiveness, particularly compared with IVF and intracytoplasmic sperm injection (ICSI).

Although the effectiveness of IUI increases in conjunction with ovarian stimulation regimens, the risk of multiple gestation is quite high with the use of gonadotropins. Less effective, clomiphene citrate is used more widely with IUI because of the relatively lower risk of multifetal gestation. Although IUI remains a common fertility treatment, it has been argued that the superiority of IVF soon will lead to discontinuation of this practice.[11]

## Reproductive Surgery

### Laparotomy

During the 1960s, fertility promoting surgeries were developed. Initially, these abdominal/pelvic operations were performed through laparotomy. Fertility surgeries were limited to salpingo-ovariolysis and salpingostomy for hydrosalpinges. Adnexal adhesions and tubal occlusion frequently resulted from sexually transmitted infections. Surgical interventions, including myomectomy, ovarian surgery, and endometriosis procedures, frequently were the cause of adnexal adhesions and resulting infertility. By the early 1970s, animal studies were able to identify several predisposing factors for adhesion formation (eg, blood/fibrin, glove talcum powder, gauze sponge trauma, saline toxicity, and ischemia). This rich trove of knowledge led to the development of reproductive microsurgery techniques.[12] The implementation of more physiologic microsurgical techniques and surgical instruments led to better surgical outcomes, translating into increased cure rates.

### Laparoscopy

Although initially used for diagnosis, it did not take long to recognize that laparoscopy provided a surgical access route as well. Advances in instrument design and the development of lightweight, high-resolution cameras enabled the expansion of operative laparoscopy for complex procedures in the late 1980s. Microsurgical techniques, including gentle tissue handling with fine instruments, remain important for fertility-promoting procedures performed at laparoscopy. Despite the improvements in laparoscopy and minimally invasive surgery, most patients with severe adhesions, endometriosis, or tubal disease do not conceive successfully following surgery. Recent improvements in IVF have led to a diminished role in these types of fertility-promoting surgeries. Anatomic problems that can have an impact on the success of IVF, such as leiomyomata and hydrosalpinges, still must be addressed. Thus, there will continue to be a role for surgery in these conditions for the foreseeable future.

### Robotic surgery

The development of the surgical robot is a major technological accomplishment. After a steep learning curve, the robot can facilitate performance of complex procedures. Despite this, the routine use of such equipment remains hotly debated. It leads to an increase in operating room and anesthesia time due to the required preparation and placement of equipment. The available evidence suggests that the use of the robot adds to the cost of laparoscopic procedures without improving measurable clinical outcomes for many surgical procedures, including tubal reconstruction.[12]

### Uterine transplantation

Many women are childless because of uncorrectable uterine disease, prior hysterectomy, or congenital absence of the uterus. Application of IVF with transfer of embryos into a gestational carrier can allow successful family building. Gestational carrier surrogacy, however, is not universally accepted due to perceived moral or ethical considerations. Many countries prohibit gestational carrier surrogacy for this reason. Uterine transplantation has been developed as an alternative. The development of this technique has been well described.[13] Studies in rodents, sheep, pigs, and baboons were required to optimize the surgical aspects, immunosuppression requirements, rejection diagnosis, and impact on pregnancy. The first successful uterine transplantation was performed on a mouse in 2003. The first birth following uterine transplantation in a woman was reported in 2014 by a Swedish team headed by Mats Brännström. In the past several years, uterine transplant programs have developed in several countries. The total number of babies born as a result of uterine transplantation remains low.[14] The procedure remains experimental and requires resolution of ethical, technical, financial, and social issues prior to widespread application. These are long and complex procedures that entail significant risk. Because immunosuppressants must be administered throughout the pregnancy with unknown long-term safety for the baby, it is unclear whether there are fewer ethical concerns than those associated with gestational carrier surrogacy.

## Fertility Medications

### Gonadotropins

In the early 1900s, animal research advanced our understanding of the pituitary and the role of gonadotropins in the control of ovulation and reproduction. In 1927, Aschheim and Zondek isolated human chorionic gonadotropin (hCG) from the urine of pregnant women.[4] Soon thereafter in 1930, Cole and Hart discovered pregnant mare serum gonadotropin. This hormone was found to have limited benefit in the treatment of infertility caused by ovulatory problems. In 1958, induction of ovulation was seen with injections of pituitary-derived gonadotropins. In 1964 Donini reported the extraction of human gonadotropins (hMGs) from human menopausal urine in sufficient quantities and later introduced the use of hMGs for ovarian stimulation as a treatment of amenorrhea. In these studies, he identified the complications of ovarian hyperstimulation syndrome (OHSS) and multiple pregnancies.

The evolution in gonadotropin technology since 1964 is a story of incremental improvements. Bioassays were developed to standardize dosing, overcoming difficulties encountered by differences in activity batch to batch. Purification processes improved to decrease the non-gonadotropin protein components, which often led to local injection reactions. Initial urinary gonadotropin preparations contained luteinizing hormone (LH) and follicle-stimulating hormone (FSH). New products were developed that eliminated the LH component. Recombinant technology was used to transition from menopausal urine to production in cultured Chinese hamster ovary cells. Modification of the carboxy terminus of the β subunit of the hCG molecule was used to produce a longer half-life and decrease dosing. Most recently, a human retinal cell line has been used to produce recombinant FSH with a glycosylation profile more similar to the human pituitary.[15]

### Oral agents to induce increased endogenous gonadotropins

Clomiphene first was synthesized in 1956 and found to be both an estrogen receptor agonist and antagonist.[4] Early animal studies suggested a contraceptive effect. The early human studies, however, demonstrated stimulation of ovulation instead of the expected suppression. The successful use of clomiphene to achieve pregnancy in a woman with anovulation was reported in 1963. Clomiphene was approved by the Food and Drug Administration (FDA) in 1967 for the indication of ovulation induction.

Other selective estrogen receptor modulators (SERMs) also have been used successfully for this purpose, including tamoxifen.[16] Additionally, aromatase inhibitors, including letrozole and anastrozole, have been used successfully as oral ovulation induction agents due to the prevention of estrogen-related gonadotropin stimulation.[17] Although letrozole has gained widespread use for ovulation induction, clomiphene remains the only drug approved by the FDA for this purpose.

Compared with gonadotropins, SERMs and aromatase inhibitors provide increased ease of use and lower risk of multifetal gestation. The disadvantage of these medications is a lower success rate, likely due to inadequate activation of estrogen receptors in the female reproductive tract.

### Assisted Reproductive Technology

IVF has evolved at a rapid pace and much of the change in fertility treatment that is predicted to occur in the next decade almost certainly will relate to optimization of IVF techniques and procedures. A historical perspective is useful to identify areas that likely will continue to evolve.

The history of mammalian IVF and embryo transfer began in Oldham, United Kingdom, in 1891, with the successful transfer of 2 fertilized eggs recovered from an Angora rabbit into the fallopian tube of a Belgian hare, producing offspring with Angora phenotypes.[18] In 1951, Min Chueh Chang and Colin Austin independently discovered capacitation, the requirement for sperm to undergo a series of surface changes in the female reproductive tract before they can fertilize the egg. This discovery paved the way for the first definitive mammalian IVF by Chang in 1959. Over the years, this success was repeated in the hamster and mouse. These studies prompted human trials by several investigators, but it was the pioneering of Robert Edwards and his colleagues in the United Kingdom that made human IVF a reality.

Edwards did not set out to treat infertility. His primary interest was the avoidance of genetic diseases like Down syndrome. It was after meeting Patrick Steptoe in 1968 that he was persuaded IVF could be a means for treating infertility. Edwards had sought out Steptoe to acquire human eggs and capacitated sperm. The need to acquire capacitated sperm from the oviduct vanished with the discovery by Barry Bavister in 1969 that capacitation of hamster eggs could be achieved simply by exposure to a raised pH.[19]

Over the next 2 years, rapid progress was made. IVF of human eggs with in vitro capacitated sperm was done in 1969. In 1971, Edwards and colleagues reported development to the blastocyst stage. From 1969 through 1978, their work was a matter of trial and error. Areas requiring optimization included ovarian stimulation, egg retrieval, sperm preparation, insemination, embryo culture, evaluation, selection, transfer, and endometrial receptivity.

Over the past 4 decades IVF, including its variants (egg donation and gestational surrogacy), has become the most successful fertility treatment. It is the primary treatment of unexplained infertility. Currently, IVF is responsible for approximately 1.9% of all babies born in the United States and its use continues to grow, having doubled in the past decade. The limiting factor for IVF utilization is affordability. In countries where IVF is provided under the national health system, such as Denmark and Israel, IVF births account for more than 5% of all births.

### DISCUSSION
#### Infertility Treatment in the Next Decade

IVF has become the dominant fertility treatment and its utilization will increase for several reasons:

1. IVF is more successful than fertility-promoting surgery and is less invasive. Although surgical technology will continue to improve incrementally, these changes will not address the underlying tubal damage or adhesion processes.
2. IVF can cure most cases of moderate to severe male factor infertility that cannot be addressed by medical or surgical approaches.
3. IVF is more successful than ovulation induction in patients with anovulation and has a much lower risk of multiple gestation.
4. Superovulation with IUI is less effective than IVF in patients with mild male factor or unexplained infertility and has a higher risk of multiple gestation.
5. Women continue to defer family building for educational and career goals. The consequences of advanced maternal age can frequently be handled through IVF with preimplantation genetic testing. Age-related ovarian failure can be addressed with egg donation.
6. Distinct from the treatment of fertility issues, IVF will become increasingly common to prevent inheritable genetic disease.

The same processes that Steptoe and Edwards had to optimize to achieve the first live birth have evolved tremendously over the past 4 decades and will continue to evolve. The next section discusses this evolution and likely future advances.

## Optimization of In Vitro Fertilization

### Ovarian stimulation
Although IVF can be performed in a natural unstimulated cycle or with minimal stimulation using oral agents, gonadotropin injections yield more eggs and embryos, thereby improving success rates.[20] Gonadotropins can cause OHSS in some patients and potentially is life-threatening. Prediction of response to gonadotropins has improved greatly through the use of sonographic antral follicle counts and serum anti-müllerian hormone (AMH) measurements. AMH correlates significantly both with risk of OHSS and IVF success.

In the late 1980s, gonadotropin-releasing hormone (GnRH) agonists were added to stimulation protocols because they increased success by decreasing the risk of premature LH surge. GnRH antagonists became available in 1999 to prevent premature ovulation while requiring fewer injections. Severe OHSS complications can be nearly eliminated when a GnRH antagonist is used to prevent ovulation and an injection of GnRH agonist is used to trigger oocyte maturation prior to egg retrieval. GnRH agonist triggers have a disadvantage of diminished endometrial receptivity, causing a lower pregnancy rate per transfer despite aggressive luteal support. This is one of the many reasons that reliance on fresh embryo transfers is decreasing and frozen embryo transfers have become dominant.[20]

Recombinant FSH preparations have not led to a complete replacement of urinary derived gonadotropins despite the advantages in production. LH activity needs to be present at threshold levels to enable the action of FSH. hMG remains widely used around the world. Additionally, FSH administration in the absence of LH/hCG activity increases the risk of premature elevations of progesterone in the follicular phase leading to embryo/endometrial asynchrony. Because of the importance of LH/hCG activity, it seems likely that a recombinant substitute for hMG that contains both recombinant FSH and recombinant hCG will be developed. The primary hurdle to approval of this type of combination gonadotropin is not scientific but rather regulatory.

### Egg retrieval
Initially, egg retrieval required laparoscopy and general anesthesia. Quickly, it was learned that this could be accomplished less invasively via ultrasound guidance.

Unlike laparoscopy, transvaginal egg retrieval does not require mechanical ventilation but rather IV sedation. This has allowed most IVF programs to transition to clinic settings.

Egg retrieval requires quality control processes to ensure that oocytes are not destroyed due to excess negative pressures. Additionally, pH and temperature should be controlled; egg collection media is prewarmed to body temperature.

Currently, follicular fluid collected in tubes is handed to an embryologist, who performs egg identification and isolation with the aid of a dissecting microscope and hand pipettes. Robotic pipetting mechanisms have become integral to many laboratory analytical instruments. It seems likely that automated systems may be engineered to perform this task of isolating eggs in the future.

### Insemination

Conventional IVF involves mixing a purified sperm sample with the isolated eggs. The first sperm that penetrates the egg initiates a cascade of events that prevents additional sperm from being able to fertilize. Importantly, in the absence of detectable sperm problems, approximately 1 in 3 eggs does not fertilize normally. Mechanical insertion of individual sperm into the egg or ICSI enables fertilization associated with severe sperm issues. ICSI initially was developed for use in male factor patients in 1992. The use of ICSI in nonmale factor infertility remains controversial, but, by 2018, 84% of IVF cycles employed ICSI rather than conventional insemination.[21]

### Embryo culture

Culture conditions are important for IVF outcome and possibly can have an impact on the future health of the offspring. Culture systems consist of culture media, protein supplements, petri dishes, and other materials as well as incubators. Handling media generally contain buffers that are able to maintain a physiologic pH outside of the incubator during egg isolation, micromanipulation, and cryopreservation. Optimal embryo culture is done in bicarbonate buffered media and hence requires high $CO_2$ concentrations (eg, 5%–6%). Many incubators also provide nitrogen to decrease the $O_2$ concentration to a more physiologic range (approximately 5%). Most frequently, an overlay of mineral or light paraffin oil is used to minimize evaporation and prevent rapid gas exchange during handling outside of the incubators.

Time-lapse incubators have been developed to allow observation of embryo development via integrated cameras. This can decrease risks associated with human handling of embryos external to the incubators. Assessment of fertilization optimally is done by observation of 2 pronuclei at 16 hours to 18 hours after insemination. This limits the time frame that both insemination and the fertilization check can be performed. These constraints are removed with time-lapse imaging. The main disadvantage to time-lapse incubators is cost. Robotic pipetting integrated into the incubator could be useful to reduce the need for skilled human embryology resources. This level of automation is not yet available. A major function of IVF incubators is to provide a warmed environment. Most laboratories set the temperature to 37°C. Mammals, however, exhibit a diurnal temperature variation as well as a shift in temperature soon after ovulation caused by progesterone. Future incubators likely may be programmed to mimic the in vivo temperature pattern.

Culture media has been greatly refined over the past 4 decades as a result of many years of animal research.[22] Initial in vitro development of rabbit embryos was described by Lewis and Gregory in 1929. Biggers achieved in vitro culture of mouse embryos in a chemically defined medium in 1962. Brinster worked on optimizing basic parameters, such as pH, osmolality, energy substrates, amino acids, and albumin, in the mid-1960s. By 1998, commercially available media was available to support routine development of human embryos to the blastocyst stage (day 5 or day 6 of culture). This was a tremendous breakthrough allowing a better ability to select embryos for transfer. Many cleavage-stage embryos stall out in development because of problems inherent to the embryo. Blastocyst transfer has a higher rate of implantation; thus, the current recommendation is to transfer only 1 blastocyst in younger women. This has resulted in a significant reduction in the risk of multiple gestation.

Despite advances, embryo culture does not precisely mimic the natural environment of the preimplantation embryo. It is likely that optimization of incubators and embryo culture media will continue for the foreseeable future.

*Cryopreservation*
As discussed previously, successful cryopreservation of human sperm first was demonstrated in 1953.[9] The technical challenge in cryopreservation of any cell is avoidance of intracellular ice crystals. Formation of these crystals can disrupt organelles and even lyse cell membranes. Sperm are the smallest cell in the human body with a large surface area–to–volume ratio. This facilitates entry of permeating cryoprotectant solutions, such as glycerol, which interacts with water molecules, thereby preventing formation of crystalline structure.

Embryos are much more susceptible to freezing injury than sperm. Whittingham and colleagues[18] published the first survival of mouse embryos producing live offspring using a slow cooling rate in the presence of the cryoprotectant dimethyl sulfoxide. The first human birth (1984) following embryo freezing used a similar slow freezing protocol. Embryo freezing technology improved over time and helped advance IVF by allowing storage of extra embryos. This helped to reduce the risk of multiple gestation and the need for repeated stimulation cycles. Over time, several other advantages were recognized, including reduction of the risk of OHSS and improved implantation rates. By 2015, the number of frozen transfers began to prevail over fresh transfers in the United States.[23]

Eggs are comparatively difficult cells to cryopreserve. They are the largest cell in the body and have a very low surface area–to–volume ratio. The difference in preservation ability also has been attributed to differences in lipid composition of cellular membranes. Occasional successful pregnancies from frozen oocytes were achieved as early as 1986 using slow freezing technique. Egg survival, however, was unpredictable, and hardening of the zona pellucida led to frequent fertilization failure. Research into oocyte cryopreservation via vitrification was accelerated by a law passed in Italy in 2004, restricting all women to the insemination of a maximum of 3 eggs, mandating the transfer of all obtained embryos, and banning embryo cryopreservation.

Vitrification is a fundamentally different approach to cryopreservation, where a sample solidifies without the formation of ice crystals, thus resulting in a glassy amorphous state. Vitrification requires higher levels of permeating cryoprotectants and a far more rapid cooling rate ($>450,000°C/min$).[24] The introduction of vitrification led to superior success rates. The routine application of ICSI for fertilization of thawed eggs was found to overcome the zona pellucida hardening issues that had long been an obstacle. In 2013, the American Society of Reproductive Medicine lifted the experimental designation applied to oocyte freezing. Vitrification of oocytes has become the standard technique for fertility preservation prior to chemotherapy for women without a male partner. Oocyte vitrification also has expanded due to many women wanting to delay family building. By 2018, more than 13,000 cycles were performed for oocyte banking for fertility preservation.[21] In general, it is recommended that egg freezing be considered before the age of 35 for optimal results. The efficient cryopreservation of eggs has also enabled the development of commercial donor egg banks.

Vitrification has also proved superior to slow freezing for blastocyst stage embryos. This process does require a higher level of embryology skills and is a cumbersome process compared with slow freezing. Because this is a manual procedure and hard to standardize, there are differences in thaw survival between embryologists. There are ongoing efforts to automate the process with robotic systems.

Currently, fertility preservation via cryopreservation of ovarian cortex remains the only process for which slow freezing maintains its edge over vitrification. Cryopreservation of ovarian tissue is the only option for fertility preservation in prepubertal girls and women who cannot delay the start of chemotherapy. After reimplantation of thawed ovarian tissue in the pelvic cavity, ovarian activity is restored in more than 95% of cases. The mean duration of ovarian function after reimplantation is 4 years to 5 years. The first pregnancy after this procedure was reported in 2004. The number of live births tallied more than 130 as of 2017. Current work centers on isolation of primordial follicles and transferring them onto a scaffold that would create an artificial ovary and avoid the need for transplantation. This will require the development of a multistep culture system to support each of the transitional stages of follicles.

### Embryo transfer

Embryo transfer is critically important for the success of IVF. Initially, the ideal conditions for embryo transfer were not known. This resulted in unnecessary complexity. Over the years, randomized studies and systematic reviews have led to standardization of the procedure.[25] The following have demonstrated importance:

- Trial, or mock, embryo transfer to map the cervical uterine anatomy, ascertain the presence of anatomic impediments, and measure the distance from the outside of the uterus to the top of the uterine cavity
- Transabdominal ultrasound guidance of soft catheters, such that the embryo placement can be visualized directly
- Inspection of the catheter post-transfer under the microscope by the embryologist to identify any retained embryos

### Preimplantation genetic testing

Robert Edwards introduced genetic testing of embryos in 1968.[17] He took biopsies from rabbit embryos and determined sex through the staining for the presence of the Barr body. Preimplantation genetic testing (PGT) was successfully put into clinical practice in 1990 with Handyside's report of birth after sex selection to avoid disease transmission by transfer of female embryos in patients with X-linked recessive disease. In 1995, the successful use of polymerase chain reaction (PCR) to avoid the transmission of Tay-Sachs disease was reported.[26] In 1995, the use of fluorescence in situ hybridization (FISH) for detection of aneuploidy was also reported.

Initially, PGT involved removal of 1 cell to 2 cells from cleavage-stage embryos. This is problematic for 2 reasons: (1) limited DNA is obtained leading to decreased test sensitivity, and (2) removal of a high proportion of the embryonic cell mass results in decreased implantation potential. In recent years, trophectoderm biopsy at the blastocyst stage has become the standard. The primary advantage of blastocyst biopsy is the ability to harvest a larger number of cells without having a significant impact on embryo viability. Most embryologists biopsy by removing cells that are spontaneously hatching from a defect created in the zona pellucida. This hole can be created mechanically or using acidic solution. The creation of a zona defect by laser generally is preferred although equipment cost remains high.

The methods of genetic testing also have evolved. FISH was prone to errors due to limited numbers of chromosomes that could be labeled at 1 time as well as frequent overlapping of chromosomes in the fixed cells that made interpretation difficult. Quantitative PCR and microarray technologies were improvements in both the sensitivity and specificity of testing. Although a broad range of methods remain, next-generation sequencing is gaining popularity due to technical advances and lower cost.

Three categories of PGT have been described: (1) PGT-M for detection of monogenic disorders, (2) PGT-SR for detection of translocations/structural rearrangements, and (3) PGT-A for detection of aneuploidy. PGT-A has become widely used in the United States to enable high success rates in conjunction with single embryo transfer. This strategy has been shown to reduce the risk of miscarriage as well as offspring with aneuploidies. The group most likely to benefit is women of advanced reproductive age. Patients should be aware that the testing is not perfect. Some genetic abnormalities are missed. Additionally, many embryos that have been tested and found abnormal have resulted in the birth of healthy offspring in cases of mosaicism.

Current research on PGT is being done with the aim of decreasing the invasiveness of the procedure by eliminating the biopsy and removal of cells. Investigations have centered on the evaluation of used embryo culture media for cell-free DNA.[27] Correlation with embryo biopsy is not yet perfect, but it is likely that these methods will be useful once optimized.

## New Disruptive Technologies

### Artificial intelligence

In medicine, imaging has been shown to benefit from application of machine learning technology. Artificial intelligence (AI) has been most widely applied in diagnostic radiology and pathology settings.[28] Advances have been made in AI embryo grading, especially at the blastocyst stage. Although contemporary embryo evaluation methods have improved, implantation rates are difficult to predict. Most advances in AI embryology are occurring with respect to embryo grading of blastocysts. Blastocyst grade has been associated with the likelihood of implantation; however, there remain significant problems, including high variability even when using time-lapse microscopy. By applying an artificial neural network using specific blastocyst features, investigators have demonstrated that an automatic morphologic classification of mouse blastocysts can be achieved with high accuracy. Retrospective analysis of human data using similar systems appears promising.[29] It seems likely that AI systems will be available soon to enhance embryo selection prior to transfer.

### Artificial gametes

Although assisted reproductive technology can be used to treat most causes of infertility, treatment of women with advanced age or patients with gonadal failure often is handled using donor gametes. This is unsatisfactory for many patients who desire genetically linked offspring.

The use of stem cell technology to create gametes shows great potential. In 2016, Hikabe and colleagues[30] reported the generation of fully potent mature oocytes from induced pluripotent stem cells derived from adult tail tip fibroblasts. Although the process is not simple, this landmark research provides a blueprint that will inspire similar work in humans. If the details can be worked out for human somatic cells, this technology could eliminate the need to obtain eggs from donors in most cases. It even is possible that eggs generated from somatic cells could eliminate the need for egg retrieval.

## SUMMARY

Treatment of infertility has evolved as understanding of reproduction has improved. Fertility promoting surgery still is performed and recent advances, including laparoscopy, robotic surgery, and uterine transplantation, continue to be refined. Hormonal treatments to correct gonadal dysfunction have been developed, but multiple gestation and associated consequences are unavoidable. Assisted reproductive technologies have been improved such that IVF and its variants increasingly are used to treat nearly all causes of infertility. Embryo cryopreservation and improved embryo selection techniques have enhanced success while lowering multiple pregnancy risk. Advances in assisted reproduction are of 2 types: (1) incremental optimization of existing techniques and (2) development of new, disruptive technologies. AI and stem cell technologies are poised to have impact in the not-so-distant future.

## CLINICS CARE POINTS

- Treatment of infertility has been considered important over millennia and across cultures.
- Surgery continues to have a role in management of some cases of infertility.
- Ovulation induction for patients with ovarian dysfunction also retains a role for anovulatory patients, but the more potent medications pose a significant risk for multifetal gestation.
- Assisted reproductive technology has seen major advances over the last four decades and plays an increasing role in the management of infertility. Further advances are likely to occur as a result of emerging stem cell technologies as well as artificial intelligence.

## DISCLOSURE

The author has no commercial or financial conflicts of interest.

## REFERENCES

1. Neto FTL, Bach PV, Lyra RJL, et al. Gods associated with male fertility and virility. Andrology 2019;7:267–72.
2. Morice P, Josset P, Chapron C, et al. History of infertility. Hum Reprod Update 1995;1(5):497–504.
3. Smith L. The Kahun gynecological papyrus: ancient Egyptian medicine. J Fam Plann Reprod Health Care 2011;37:54–5.
4. Beall S, Decherney A. The history and challenges surrounding ovarian stimulation in the treatment of infertility. Fertil Steril 2012;97(4):795–801.
5. Howards S. Antoine van Leeuwenhoek and the discovery of sperm. Fert Steril 1997;67(1):16–7.
6. Ombelet W, Van Robays J. Artificial insemination history: hurdles and milestones. Facts Views Vis Obgyn 2015;7(2):137–43.
7. Guttmacher AF. The role of artificial insemination in the treatment of human sterility. Bull N Y Acad Med 1943;19(8):573–9.
8. Polge C, Smith A, Parkes A. Revival of spermatozoa after vitrification and dehydration at low temperatures. Nature 1949;164:66.
9. Sztein JM, Takeo T, Nakagata N. History of cryobiology, with special emphasis in evolution of mouse sperm cryopreservation. Cryobiology 2018;82:57–63.

10. Byrd W, Ackerman GE, Carr BR, et al. Treatment of refractory infertility by trans-cervical intrauterine insemination of washed spermatatozoa. Fertil Steril 1987; 48(6):921–7.
11. Ombelet W, van Eekelen R, McNally A, et al. Should couples with unexplained infertility have three to six cycles of intrauterine insemination with ovarian stimulation or in vitro fertilization as first-line treatment. Fertil Steril 2020;114(6):1141–8.
12. Gomel V. From laparotomy to laparoscopy to in vitro fertilization. Fertil Steril 2019; 112(2):183–96.
13. Castellon LAR, Amador MIG, Gonzalez RED, et al. The history behind successful uterine transplantation in humans. JBRA Assist Reprod 2017;21:126–34.
14. Gomel V. Uterine transplantation. Climacteric 2019;22(2):117–21.
15. Olsson H, Sandstrom R, Grundemar L. Different pharmacokinetic and pharmacodynamic properties of recombinant follicle-stimulating hormone (rFSH) derived from a human cell line compared with rFSH from a non-human cell line. J Clin Pharmacol 2014;54(11):1299–307.
16. Messinis IE, Nillius SJ. Comparison between tamoxifen and clomiphene for induction of ovulation. Acta Obstet Gynecol Scand 1982;61(4):377–9.
17. Mitwally MF, Biljan MM, Casper RF. Pregnancy outcome after the use of an aromatase inhibitor for ovarian stimulation. Am J Obstet Gynecol 2005;192(2):381–6.
18. Johnson M. Human in vitro fertilization and developmental biology: a mutually influential history. Development 2019;146(17):dev183145.
19. Fishel S. First in vitro fertilization baby- this is how it happened. Fertil Steril 2018; 110(1):5–11.
20. Eskew AM, Jungheim ES. A history of developments to improve in vitro fertilization. Mo Med May 2017;114(3):156–9.
21. National summary report. SART; 2018. Available at: https://www.sartcorsonline.com/rptCSR_PublicMultYear.aspx?reportingYear=2018.
22. Chronopoulou E, Harper JC. IVF culture media: past, present, and future. Hum Reprod Update 2015;21(1):9–55.
23. De Geyter CH, Wyns C, Calhaz-Jorge C, et al. 20 years of the European ivf-monitoring consortium registry: what have we learned? A comparison with registries from two other regions. Hum Reprod 2020;35(12):2832–49.
24. Arav A, Natan Y. The near future of vitrification of oocytes and embryos: looking into past experience and planning into the future. Transfus Med Hemother 2019; 46:182–6.
25. Practice Committee of the American Society for Reproductive Medicine. ASRM standard embryo transfer protocol template: a committee opinion. Fertil Steril 2017;107(4):897–900.
26. Takeuchi K. Pre-implantation genetic testing: past, present, future. Reprod Med Biol 2021;20:27–40.
27. Shitara A, Takahashi K, Goto M, et al. Cell-free DNA in spent culture medium effectively reflects the chromosomal status of embryos following culturing beyond implantation compared to trophectoderm biopsy. PLoS One 2021;16(2):1–13.
28. Zaninovic N, Rosenwaks Z. Artificial intelligence in human in vitro fertilization and embryology. Fertil Steril 2020;114(5):914–20.
29. VerMilyea M, Hall JMM, Diakiw SM, et al. Development of an artificial intelligence-based assessment model for prediction of embryo viability using static images captured by optical light microscopy during IVF. Hum Reprod 2020;35(4):770–84.
30. Hikabe O, Hamazaki N, Nagamatsu G, et al. Reconstitution in vitro of the entire cycle of the mouse female germ line. Nature 2016;539:299.

# Postscript
## Women's Health and the Era After COVID-19

Denisse S. Holcomb, MD[a],*, William F. Rayburn, MD, MBA[b]

### KEYWORDS

- COVID-19 • Future • Medical education • Obstetrics & gynecology
- Practice change • Safety • Telehealth • Vaccinations

### KEY POINTS

- Disruptive changes from the COVID-19 pandemic has led to a heightened focus on safety in the office, on labor and delivery, and in the operating room.
- Greater utilization of telehealth has gained more acceptance in all aspects of women's health care.
- The lack of pregnant and lactating women enrolled in COVID-19 clinical trials has raised public concerns.
- Virtual meetings are common and have led to significant changes in patient care and education delivery.
- More attention toward marginalized communities and needs of the diverse women's health care workforce will create opportunities for improvement.

*You can't solve a problem in the same level that it was created. You have to rise above it to the next level.*
—*Albert Einstein*

### INTRODUCTION

This issue of the *Obstetrics and Gynecology Clinics of North America* was planned in 2019 before the emergence of the coronavirus disease 2019 (COVID-19) in December 2019 in the Hubei Province, China.[1] As COVID-19 was declared a pandemic by the World Health Organization on March 11, 2020, health care systems were required to rapidly adapt given safety concerns for both patients and health care personnel. In the field of obstetrics and gynecology, these concerns led to the postponement of well-women visits, adjustments of the prenatal and postpartum visit schedule, implementation of telehealth visits, cancellation of elective gynecologic surgeries, patient symptom prescreening before visits, and other adaptations.[2–4]

---

[a] Department of Obstetrics and Gynecology, University of Texas Southwestern Center, Dallas, TX, USA; [b] Department of Obstetrics and Gynecology, University of New Mexico School of Medicine, Albuquerque, NM, USA
* Corresponding author. 5939 Harry Hines Boulevard, Dallas, TX 75390.
*E-mail address:* denisse.holcomb@utsouthwestern.edu

Obstet Gynecol Clin N Am 48 (2021) 813–821
https://doi.org/10.1016/j.ogc.2021.06.002     obgyn.theclinics.com
0889-8545/21/© 2021 Elsevier Inc. All rights reserved.

In response to changes resulting from the pandemic, the authors elected to end this issue with a commentary on lessons learned that may impact the future of our specialty. We do not claim to be experts, but we did endure this experience while providing patient care. Preparing this postscript created an opportunity to reflect, add perspective, and begin to navigate several directions from this experience that would affect the future of our practices.

## CHANGES IN OUTPATIENT SETTINGS
### Abbreviating the Prenatal Schedule

Precautions about minimizing direct exposure to potentially infected patients prompted a reevaluation of the conventional prenatal visit schedule comprised of 12 to 14 visits.[3,5,6] Throughout the country, obstetricians have adopted either abbreviated or hybrid schedules, comprised of both in-person and telehealth visits. This pandemic-shifted paradigm from the traditional prenatal schedule has been endorsed by American College of Obstetricians and Gynecologists (ACOG). Although a revision of this standard prenatal schedule has long been overdue and supported by numerous studies, it took a worldwide pandemic to prompt change.[7–9] Since implementation, many groups have documented patient support of these changes. As society continues to conform to decreased in-person visits, it is difficult to imagine a world where this is reverted following the COVID-19 pandemic. The authors anticipate that this rightsizing of maternity care will continue in the postpartum period that may extend to a 12-month period.

### Telehealth

In response to COVID-19, obstetrician and gynecologist (ob-gyn) practices rapidly adapted by quickly implementing telehealth visits. Publication of the *Obstetrics and Gynecology Clinics of North America* issue pertaining to telehealth in obstetrics and gynecology (Telemedicine and Connected Health in Obstetrics and Gynecology, *Obstet Gynecol Clin*, volume 42.2, June 2020) was well timed. Interim measures by the Centers for Medicare and Medicaid Services (CMS) and the Department of Health and Human Services helped decrease barriers to the speedy adoption of telehealth services.[10,11] Physicians suddenly found themselves able to see new patients via telehealth, provide audio-only visits when most convenient to patients, get reimbursed for these visits at the same rates as in-person visits, and see patients across state lines without barriers.[11,12] Longer-term policies adopted by CMS and across all payors will be essential to allow this improved access to care and thus help reduce travel, especially from rural locations.

### Outpatient Gynecology

As the pandemic commenced in the United States, attention focused on limiting outpatient clinic visits. Gynecologists quickly had to consider how to prevent barriers to contraception in this new paradigm. ACOG quickly provided guidance on the use of telehealth visits for contraceptive counseling and prescribing; they also recommended filling contraceptives for a full year and to consider proactively prescribing emergency contraception to those patients that desired it.[4] ACOG also recommended that long acting reversible contraception (LARC) methods continue to be offered. It remains to be seen what the long-term effects of such strategies are.

### Mental Health

The COVID-19 pandemic has had a great impact on patients in myriad ways. Social isolation, economic hardship, limited resources, uncertainty of the future, and illness or even death of close family members are all factors that have contributed to the nearly 3-fold higher prevalence of depression symptoms noted in the United States as compared with the pre-COVID era.[13] As we continue to move past this pandemic, we must remember to address both the physical and the emotional needs of our patients to improve recognition of potential mental illness. Health care systems and professional organizations will need to come up with innovative ways to increase access to mental health resources for all patients in order to meet the increasing demand.

## CHANGES IN HOSPITAL SETTINGS
### Labor and Delivery

The labor and delivery (L&D) unit is the most frequent site for direct hospitalization in obstetrics. As L&Ds throughout the country struggled to keep up with steady obstetric volumes despite quarantine efforts and social distancing mandates, attention was directed at maintaining a safe environment for both patients and hospital personnel. From employee and patient screening efforts, use of personal protection equipment (PPE) for hospital personnel, universal mask mandates for patients and visitors, and universal COVID-19 testing for patients in labor, we have learned a great deal about infectious disease transmission best practices.[14,15] Those practices developed during the past 2 years will continue in some ways. Visitors will likely continue to be limited, and some form of universal infection screening will persist despite many persons being asymptomatic. Vigilant use of PPE, performance of frequent handwashing, and universal precautions will likely continue more than before the pandemic.

### Gynecology

The COVID-19 pandemic led to recommendations that nonemergent elective medical and surgical services be canceled or delayed, to reduce exposures and allow for preservation of PPE for emergency procedures.[16,17] National guidance prompted hospitals to adopt universal preoperative COVID-19 testing to allow for extra protective measures used during aerosolizing procedures in the event of COVID-19 exposure. As the number of cases slowly declined and PPE manufacturing continued to improve, resumption of elective surgical procedures commenced. We expect an uptick of gynecologic cases as patients return to their gynecologists. As we move forward past this pandemic, we suspect that presurgical screening for infectious disease will remain.

## MEDICAL EDUCATION

The COVID-19 pandemic has dramatically impacted the educational experience for trainees at all levels. For medical students, opportunities for direct patient care were placed at a standstill to preserve precious PPE.[18] Didactic sessions became virtual (live or recorded), and small group teaching was limited because of the absence of patient assignments. An assessment from this lack of direct patient contact will be necessary to determine whether a student's knowledge base was undermined as a result. The interview process for students applying for obstetrics and gynecology residencies was converted to virtual experiences to reduce exposure to potentially infected individuals. As the COVID-19 pandemic recedes, we should consider whether residency interviews should remain virtual, given its advantages, such as reduced cost and decreased time away from elective courses.

The importance of resident and fellow safety, supervision, and work hour requirements will continue to be closely scrutinized.[19] Lessons were learned from the COVID-19 experience about team building and interprofessional education. Any impact on suspending normal block rotations and deploying residents and fellows to cover obstetric services and urgent gynecologic cases will warrant examination. Close attention will need to be paid to the impact of suspending elective surgical procedures on resident surgical experience and education. As graduating residents join practices, postgraduate training workshops and seminars in addition to targeted mentorship programs may help provide support for this cohort of obstetrician/gynecologists as they enter the workforce.

Virtual conferences, rather than onsite regional or national meetings, are likely to remain as a popular option. Some hybrids of virtual learning (synchronous and asynchronous) with in-person teaching will be necessary, bringing both benefits and challenges. The mode of delivery will depend on the educational activity to address the practical needs of learners to better close their knowledge gap and improve their performance. Furthermore, special attention should be paid to provide training in telemedicine for trainees of all levels, as this is most likely to remain substantial means of health care delivery.[20]

Although unclear at this time, it will be interesting to discover how the American Board of Obstetrics and Gynecology will alter its approach to certification and recertification of graduating ob-gyn residents and those in practice. Whether the COVID-19 pandemic will affect the timing and administration of written and oral examinations and collection of cases remains to be seen. The requirement of answering questions pertaining to select medical journal articles will probably remain a popular means of focused learning at the home or office for continuing education credit.

## RESEARCH
### Research in Women's Health

Viral infection outbreaks from the HIV, Zika, and COVID-19 prompted needs for immediate and long-term research that impacted women's health. More unique to the coronavirus pandemic was social distancing, with many research activities being suspended early.[21] Reduced productivity was seen. Research meetings became mostly virtual, and many national scientific organizations either canceled their in-person meetings or replaced them with virtual meetings. As we move past this pandemic, it is likely that virtual meetings as a mode for data exchange will persist. Furthermore, lessons were learned during COVID-19 about the need for research practices to be prompter and more nationwide.

### Coronavirus 2019 Vaccination Trials

The COVID-19 pandemic shed light on the everyday exclusion of pregnant and lactating women in clinical trials of therapeutics and vaccines, prompting uncertainty in counseling patients.[22] At the time of publication, Whitehead and Walker[22] reported nearly universal exclusion of pregnant women from more than 300 trials for COVID-19 treatments. Even before this pandemic, infectious diseases like Zika and HIV virus have placed the practice of excluding pregnant women into question.[23] In 2016, the Task Force on Research Specific to Pregnant Women and Lactating Women provided a proactive protocol to allow for the safe inclusion of pregnant and breastfeeding women in clinical trials.[24] Several years later, this pandemic has provided us with yet another example of the consequences of such exclusions.

As numerous pharmaceutical companies early in the pandemic joined the race for COVID-19 vaccination Food and Drug Administration (FDA) authorization, it became clear that pregnant and lactating women were being excluded. Despite the paucity of data on the current FDA-authorized vaccines available, ACOG, the Society for Maternal Fetal Medicine, and the Centers for Disease Control and Prevention (CDC) recommended that the COVID-19 vaccines not be withheld from pregnant or lactating women who meet criteria for vaccination based on the Advisory Council for Immunization Practices recommendations.[25,26] Minimal data from animal studies on messenger RNA vaccines and inadvertently vaccinated pregnant people have demonstrated no harmful effects.[27,28] Since the FDA began to issue emergency use authorizations to pharmaceutical companies for COVID-19 vaccines,[28,29] we have had to counsel our patients through a process of shared decision making, citing the limited data available as well as the science basis for vaccine efficacy and potential harms of being infected during pregnancy. As the Pfizer COVID-19 vaccine undertakes a global clinical trial on pregnant women in the upcoming year, perhaps other drug companies will follow suit.[30]

## SERVICE TO AT-RISK AND MARGINALIZED COMMUNITIES

Responses during the COVID-19 crisis affected all communities, particularly those already experiencing structural, societal, economic, and health inequities. From the onset of the pandemic, health disparities were noted for those locations that reported data on race and ethnicity, with African Americans and Latinos carrying a disproportionate burden of adverse outcomes.[31] Reasons for these inequalities are likely multifaceted, including social determinants of health, racism, discrimination, economic disadvantages, health care access, and preexisting comorbidities.[32]

Interest in diversity, equity, and inclusiveness has accelerated a culture of belongingness and inclusiveness over the past 2 years. The pandemic should encourage the development of government-sponsored registries in the collection, evaluation, and reporting of COVID-19–specific data, including race and ethnicity. These data would aid in understanding of whether infection-induced morbidity and mortality relate to economic or racial inequities in maternal health access, preventive services including contraception, and health outcomes. Planning and prioritization of resources can thus result from evaluating crisis responses on marginalized communities. Innovative solutions to promote the health of incarcerated, emotionally challenged, or homeless people and to avoid suspension of medically inappropriate restrictions may arise from the COVID-19 experience.

## INVESTING IN THE WOMEN'S HEALTH WORKFORCE

Like all physicians, particularly those who were procedure based, ob-gyns had reductions in revenue production as elective surgeries, office visits, and staff availability declined early during the pandemic.[33] New and existing financial relief programs are important and require periodic examination.[34] Medicaid physicians need support through appropriate reimbursement, including maternity care and participation by all willing and qualified providers. Equitable reimbursement and coverage are necessary to scale-up ob-gyn's telehealth use for essential health services, such as prenatal and postpartum physical and mental health services.

Expansion of physician license portability and multistate licensure privileges would be appropriate to consider more seriously. Liability of health care professionals needed to be protected in providing services within the scope of authority under COVID-19 emergency. This could expand to other conditions and circumstances associated with the public health emergencies.[35] As safer working conditions continue, protection from retaliation for reporting unsafe practices are necessary to support health care professionals.

The pandemic has weighed emotionally on most health care workers throughout the country. Long work hours, PPE shortages, increased patient deaths in hospitals, fear of infecting loved ones, and decisions on reallocation of health resources have contributed to psychological stressors that all physicians have faced.[36] As we move past this pandemic, we must remember to address what our workforce has endured to allow for rebuilding and healing. Education on psychosocial issues during COVID-19 should be provided to not only patients but also health care workers by professional organizations and health systems alike.

Obstetrics and gynecology has the highest proportion of female physicians. The COVID-19 pandemic has further impacted the balance of household duties and child-care that disproportionately fall on female health care professionals compared with their male colleagues. This was particularly pronounced when the country's K-12 education was largely accessible only through virtual learning at home.[37] The stress of advancing professionally and practicing, while attempting to meet the emotional and educational needs of their children, created significant professional and personal conflicts and impacted further on any burnout. For ob-gyn faculty, an understanding and the support from their department chairs and division directors are necessary in making accommodations to ensure an appropriate work-life balance that does not significantly derail academic career development.[38,39] An opportunity exists for academic and community departments of obstetrics and gynecology to take a lead in developing innovative strategies and serve as role models to handle these fundamental changes now and in the future.

## ETHICAL CONSIDERATIONS

As the COVID-19 pandemic evolved, ob-gyns faced numerous ethical questions related to how they would practice within the social and political confines of our country. Early on, patients often received conflicting information about the coronavirus and would turn to their physicians for further guidance. Physicians, in turn, had to quickly modify their existing patient care infrastructures to meet the demands of a newly evolving pandemic. Even when expert opinion and guidance were provided from the CDC, there still existed a lack of information on how to optimize patient care in the context of COVID-19.

---

**Box 1**
**Ethical questions affecting obstetricians and gynecologists during the COVID-19 pandemic**

How can ob-gyns navigate the competing interests of providing the best care for individual patients with the responsibility of safeguarding public health?

What principles can help health care systems allocate limited health care resources?

What are the ethical considerations and implications of postponing nonurgent surgical procedures and clinic visits?

What are the ethical considerations associated with caring for patients without adequate PPE available?

How can ob-gyns maintain rapport with patients through telehealth?

What are ethical considerations regarding enrolling pregnant patients in vaccinations trials for COVID-19?

What are ethical considerations in caring for patients who refuse preprocedure COVID-19 testing?

*Data from* American College of Obstetricians and Gynecologists. COVID-19 FAQs for obstetricians-gynecologists, ethics. Washington, DC: ACOG; 2020.

This rapidly evolving situation led to the development of protocols that attempted to meet the health care needs of patients. Frequently ethical dilemmas were also encountered. Examples of frequently asked questions to ACOG, as shown in **Box 1**, required frequent updated responses.[40] As we move past the COVID-19 pandemic, ob-gyns will have gained knowledge on how to balance patient care and public safety simultaneously. We will also feel better prepared to respond to such ethical dilemmas that may be encountered in future public health emergencies.

## SUMMARY

Despite the challenges faced by women's health care communities during the COVID-19 pandemic, we will continue to meet the needs of our patients and families. Every health care organization faces crises at one time or another, but the ones who weather them best have a clear sense of mission, have strong leadership in place, and communicate regularly with staff, patients, and the community throughout the pandemic. As a second year of transition draws to a close, we encourage you and your health care team to take the opportunity to pause, reflect, and appreciate the important contributions you have made. A commitment to change during and after this shift to a "new normal" will require outcome measures. Lessons learned from this pandemic in patient care, medical education, technology and clinical research, marginalized communities, and our workforce will serve us in accelerating efforts to provide high-quality care to our patients and fulfillment to our profession.

## DISCLOSURE

The authors have no financial disclosures or conflicts of interest to report.

## REFERENCES

1. World Health Organization. Timeline: WHO's COVID-19 response. Available at: https://www.who.int/emergencies/diseases/novel-coronavirus-2019/interactive-timeline/#!. Accessed February 28, 2021.
2. American College of Obstetricians and Gynecologists. Novel coronavirus 2019 (COVID-19) practice advisory. Available at: https://www.acog.org/clinical/clinical-guidance/practice-advisory/articles/2020/03/novel-coronavirus-2019. Accessed February 28, 2021.
3. American College of Obstetricians and Gynecologists. COVID-19 FAQs for obstetrician-gynecologists, obstetrics. Available at: https://www.acog.org/clinical-information/physician-faqs/covid-19-faqs-for-ob-gyns-obstetrics. Accessed February 24, 2021.
4. American College of Obstetricians and Gynecologists. COVID-19 FAQs for obstetrician-gynecologists, gynecology. Available at: https://www.acog.org/clinical-information/physician-faqs/covid19-faqs-for-ob-gyns-gynecology. Accessed February 24, 2021.
5. Peahl AF, Smith RD, Moniz MH. Prenatal care redesign: creating flexible maternity care models through virtual care. Am J Obstet Gynecol 2020;223(3):389.e1–10.
6. Duzyj CM, Thornburg LL, Han CS. Practice modification for pandemics. Obstet Gynecol 2020;136(2):237–51.
7. Peahl AF, Heisler M, Essenmacher LK, et al. A comparison of international prenatal care guidelines for low-risk women to inform high-value care. Am J Obstet Gynecol 2020;222:505–7.

8. Dowswell T, Carroli G, Duley L, et al. Alternative versus standard packages of antenatal care for low-risk pregnancy. Cochrane Database Syst Rev 2015; 2015:CD000934.

9. Butler Tobah YS, LeBlanc A, Branda ME, et al. Randomized comparison of a reduced-visit prenatal care model enhanced with remote monitoring. Am J Obstet Gynecol 2019;221:638. e1-8.

10. Centers for Medicare & Medicaid Services. Medicare telemedicine health care provider fact sheet. Available at: https://www.cms.gov/newsroom/fact-sheets/medicare-telemedicine-health-care-provider-fact-sheet. Accessed February 23, 2021.

11. U.S. Department of Health and Human Services Office for Civil Rights (OCR). Notification of enforcement discretion for telehealth remote communications during the COVID-19 nationwide public health emergency. Available at: https://www.hhs.gov/hipaa/for-professionals/special-topics/emergency-preparedness/notification-enforcement-discretion-telehealth/index.html. Accessed February 23, 2021.

12. Wosik J, Fudim M, Cameron B, et al. Telehealth transformation: COVID-19 and the rise of virtual care. J Am Med Inform Assoc 2020;27(6):957–62.

13. Ettman CK, Abdalla SM, Cohen GH, et al. Prevalence of depression symptoms in US adults before and during the COVID-19 pandemic. JAMA Netw Open 2020; 3(9):e2019686.

14. Sutton D, Fuchs K, D'Alton M, et al. Universal screening for SARS-CoV-2 in women admitted for delivery. N Engl J Med 2020;382:2163–4.

15. Jamieson DJ, Steinberg JP, Martinello RA, et al. Obstetricians on the coronavirus disease 2019 (COVID-19) front lines and the confusing world of personal protective equipment. Obstet Gynecol 2020;135:1257–63.

16. CMS. Non-emergent, elective medical services, and treatment recommendations. Available at: https://www.cms.gov/files/document/cms-non-emergent-elective-medical-recommendations.pdf. Accessed February 25, 2021.

17. American College of Surgeons Joint statement: road map for resuming elective surgery after COVID-19 pandemic. Available at: https://www.facs.org/covid-19/clinical-guidance/roadmap-elective-surgery. Accessed February 25, 2021.

18. Rose S. Medical student education in the time of COVID-19. JAMA 2020;323(21): 2131–2.

19. Accreditation Council for Graduate Medical Education. ACGME resident/fellow education and training considerations related to coronavirus (COVID-19). Available at: https://www.acgme.org/Newsroom/Newsroom-Details/ArticleID/10085/ACGME-Resident-Fellow-Education-and-Training-Considerations-related-to-Coronavirus-COVID-19. Accessed February 28, 2021.

20. Edirippulige S, Armfield NR. Education and training to support the use of clinical telehealth: a review of the literature. J Telemed Telecare 2017;23(2):273–82.

21. Alvarez RD, Goff BA, Chelmow D, et al. Reengineering academic departments of obstetrics and gynecology to operate in a pandemic world and beyond: a joint American Gynecological and Obstetrical Society and Council of University Chairs of Obstetrics and Gynecology statement. Am J Obstet Gynecol 2020;223:383–8.

22. Whitehead CL, Walker SP. Consider pregnancy in COVID-19 therapeutic drug and vaccine trials. Lancet 2020;395(10237):e92.

23. Cohen J. Zika rewrites maternal immunization ethics. Science 2017; 357(6348):241.

24. Eunice Kennedy Shriver National Institute of Child Health and Human Development. Task force on research specific to pregnant women and lactating women

(PRGLAC). December 29. 2020. Available at: https://www.nichd.nih.gov/about/advisory/PRGLAC. Accessed February 24, 2021.

25. Centers for Disease Control and Prevention. Vaccination considerations for people who are pregnant or breastfeeding. Available at: https://www-cdc-gov.libproxy.unm.edu/coronavirus/2019-ncov/vaccines/recommendations/pregnancy.html. Accessed February 20, 2021.

26. American College of Obstetricians and Gynecologists. Practice advisory. Vaccinating pregnant and lactating patients against COVID-19. Available at: https://www.acog.org/clinical/clinical-guidance/practice-advisory/articles/2020/12/vaccinating-pregnant-and-lactating-patients-against-covid-19. Accessed February 27, 2021.

27. Dashraath P, Nielsen-Saines K, Madhi SA, et al. COVID-19 vaccines and neglected pregnancy. Lancet 2020;396(10252):e22.

28. FDA. Emergency use authorization (EUA). Pfizer-BioNTech COVID-19 vaccine/BNT162b2. Available at: https://www-fda-gov.libproxy.unm.edu/emergency-preparedness-and-response/coronavirus-disease-2019-covid-19/pfizer-biontech-covid-19-vaccine. Accessed February 25, 2021.

29. Emergency Use Authorization (EUA). Moderna COVID-19 vaccine/mRNA-1273. Available at: https://www-fda-gov.libproxy.unm.edu/emergency-preparedness-and-response/coronavirus-disease-2019-covid-19/moderna-covid-19-vaccine. Accessed February 25, 2021.

30. Pfizer. Pfizer and Biontech commence global clinical trial to evaluate COVID-19 vaccine in pregnant women. Available at: https://www.pfizer.com/news/press-release/press-release-detail/pfizer-and-biontech-commence-global-clinical-trial-evaluate. Accessed February 28, 2021.

31. Webb Hooper M, Nápoles AM, Pérez-Stable EJ. COVID-19 and racial/ethnic disparities. JAMA 2020 23;323(24):2466–7.

32. Yancy CW. COVID-19 and African Americans. JAMA 2020;323(19):1891–2.

33. Rubin R. COVID-19's crushing effects on medical practices, some of which might not survive. JAMA 2020;324(4):321–3.

34. American College of Obstetricians and Gynecologists. Financial support for physicians and practices during the COVID-19 pandemic. Available at: https://www.acog.org/practice-management/payment-resources/resources/financial-support-for-physicians-and-practices-during-the-covid-19-pandemic. Accessed February 28, 2021.

35. CMS. COVID-19 emergency declaration blanket waivers for health care providers. Available at: https://www.cms.gov/files/document/summary-covid-19-emergency-declaration-waivers.pdf. Accessed February 28, 2021.

36. Pfefferbaum B, North CS. Mental health and the Covid-19 pandemic. N Engl J Med 2020;383(6):510–2.

37. Black E, Ferdig R, Thompson LA. K-12 virtual schooling, COVID-19, and student success. JAMA Pediatr 2021;175(2):119–20.

38. Gabster BP, van Daalen K, Khatt R, et al. Challenges for the female academic during the COVID-19 pandemic. Lancet 2020;395:1968–70.

39. Brubaker L. Women physicians and the COVID-19 pandemic. JAMA 2020;324:835–6.

40. American College of Obstetricians and Gynecologists. COVID-19 FAQs for obstetricians-gynecologists, ethics. Washington, DC: ACOG; 2020. Available at: https://www.acog.org/clinical-information/physician-faqs/covid-19-faqs-for-ob-gyns-ethics. Accessed February 24, 2021.

# UNITED STATES POSTAL SERVICE® Statement of Ownership, Management, and Circulation (All Periodicals Publications Except Requester Publications)

| 1. Publication Title | 2. Publication Number | 3. Filing Date |
|---|---|---|
| OBSTETRICS AND GYNECOLOGY CLINICS OF NORTH AMERICA | 000 – 276 | 9/18/2021 |

| 4. Issue Frequency | 5. Number of Issues Published Annually | 6. Annual Subscription Price |
|---|---|---|
| MAR, JUN, SEP, DEC | 4 | $335.00 |

7. Complete Mailing Address of Known Office of Publication (Not printer) (Street, city, county, state, and ZIP+4®)

ELSEVIER INC.
230 Park Avenue, Suite 800
New York, NY 10169

Contact Person
Malathi Samayan

Telephone (Include area code)
91-44-4299-4507

8. Complete Mailing Address of Headquarters or General Business Office of Publisher (Not printer)

ELSEVIER INC.
230 Park Avenue, Suite 800
New York, NY 10169

9. Full Names and Complete Mailing Addresses of Publisher, Editor, and Managing Editor (Do not leave blank)

Publisher (Name and complete mailing address)

Editor (Name and complete mailing address)

KERRY HOLLAND, ELSEVIER INC.
1600 JOHN F KENNEDY BLVD. SUITE 1800
PHILADELPHIA, PA 19103-2899

Managing Editor (Name and complete mailing address)

PATRICK MANLEY, ELSEVIER INC.
1600 JOHN F KENNEDY BLVD. SUITE 1800
PHILADELPHIA, PA 19103-2899

10. Owner (Do not leave blank. If the publication is owned by a corporation, give the name and address of the corporation immediately followed by the names and addresses of all stockholders owning or holding 1 percent or more of the total amount of stock. If not owned by a corporation, give the names and addresses of the individual owners. If owned by a partnership or other unincorporated firm, give its name and address as well as those of each individual owner. If the publication is published by a nonprofit organization, give its name and address.)

| Full Name | Complete Mailing Address |
|---|---|
| WHOLLY OWNED SUBSIDIARY OF REED/ELSEVIER, US HOLDINGS | 1600 JOHN F KENNEDY BLVD. SUITE 1800 PHILADELPHIA, PA 19103-2899 |

11. Known Bondholders, Mortgagees, and Other Security Holders Owning or Holding 1 Percent or More of Total Amount of Bonds, Mortgages, or Other Securities. If none, check box ▸ ☐ None

| Full Name | Complete Mailing Address |
|---|---|
| N/A | |

12. Tax Status (For completion by nonprofit organizations authorized to mail at nonprofit rates) (Check one)
The purpose, function, and nonprofit status of this organization and the exempt status for federal income tax purposes:
☒ Has Not Changed During Preceding 12 Months
☐ Has Changed During Preceding 12 Months (Publisher must submit explanation of change with this statement)

PS Form **3526**, July 2014 (Page 1 of 4 (see instructions page 4)) PSN: 7530-01-000-9931 PRIVACY NOTICE: See our privacy policy on www.usps.com.

| 13. Publication Title | 14. Issue Date for Circulation Data Below |
|---|---|
| OBSTETRICS AND GYNECOLOGY CLINICS OF NORTH AMERICA | JUNE 2021 |

| 15. Extent and Nature of Circulation | | Average No. Copies Each Issue During Preceding 12 Months | No. Copies of Single Issue Published Nearest to Filing Date |
|---|---|---|---|
| a. Total Number of Copies (Net press run) | | 215 | 172 |
| b. Paid Circulation (By Mail and Outside the Mail) | (1) Mailed Outside-County Paid Subscriptions Stated on PS Form 3541 (Include paid distribution above nominal rate, advertiser's proof copies, and exchange copies) | 54 | 45 |
| | (2) Mailed In-County Paid Subscriptions Stated on PS Form 3541 (Include paid distribution above nominal rate, advertiser's proof copies, and exchange copies) | 0 | 0 |
| | (3) Paid Distribution Outside the Mails Including Sales Through Dealers and Carriers, Street Vendors, Counter Sales, and Other Paid Distribution Outside USPS® | 109 | 91 |
| | (4) Paid Distribution by Other Classes of Mail Through the USPS (e.g., First-Class Mail®) | 0 | 0 |
| c. Total Paid Distribution (Sum of 15b (1), (2), (3), and (4)) | | 163 | 136 |
| d. Free or Nominal Rate Distribution (By Mail and Outside the Mail) | (1) Free or Nominal Rate Outside-County Copies Included on PS Form 3541 | 34 | 17 |
| | (2) Free or Nominal Rate In-County Copies Included on PS Form 3541 | 0 | 0 |
| | (3) Free or Nominal Rate Copies Mailed at Other Classes Through the USPS (e.g., First-Class Mail) | 0 | 0 |
| | (4) Free or Nominal Rate Distribution Outside the Mail (Carriers or other means) | 34 | 17 |
| e. Total Free or Nominal Rate Distribution (Sum of 15d (1), (2), (3) and (4)) | | 34 | 17 |
| f. Total Distribution (Sum of 15c and 15e) | | 197 | 153 |
| g. Copies not Distributed (See Instructions to Publishers #4 (page #3)) | | 18 | 19 |
| h. Total (Sum of 15f and g) | | 215 | 172 |
| i. Percent Paid (15c divided by 15f times 100) | | 82.74% | 88.89% |

* If you are claiming electronic copies, go to line 16 on page 3. If you are not claiming electronic copies, skip to line 17 on page 3.

| 16. Electronic Copy Circulation | | Average No. Copies Each Issue During Preceding 12 Months | No. Copies of Single Issue Published Nearest to Filing Date |
|---|---|---|---|
| a. Paid Electronic Copies | ▸ | | |
| b. Total Paid Print Copies (Line 15c) + Paid Electronic Copies (Line 16a) | ▸ | | |
| c. Total Print Distribution (Line 15f) + Paid Electronic Copies (Line 16a) | ▸ | | |
| d. Percent Paid (Both Print & Electronic Copies) (16b divided by 16c × 100) | ▸ | | |

☒ I certify that 50% of all my distributed copies (electronic and print) are paid above a nominal prices.

17. Publication of Statement of Ownership

☒ If the publication is a general publication, publication of this statement is required. Will be printed ☐ Publication not required
in the DECEMBER 2021 issue of this publication.

18. Signature and Title of Editor, Publisher, Business Manager, or Owner

Malathi Samayan - Distribution Controller

*Malathi Samayan*

Date 9/18/2021

I certify that all information furnished on this form is true and complete. I understand that anyone who furnishes false or misleading information on this form or who omits material or information requested on the form may be subject to criminal sanctions (including fines and imprisonment) and/or civil sanctions (including civil penalties).

PS Form **3526**, July 2014 (Page 3 of 4) PRIVACY NOTICE: See our privacy policy on www.usps.com

# Moving?

## Make sure your subscription moves with you!

To notify us of your new address, find your **Clinics Account Number** (located on your mailing label above your name), and contact customer service at:

Email: **journalscustomerservice-usa@elsevier.com**

**800-654-2452** (subscribers in the U.S. & Canada)
**314-447-8871** (subscribers outside of the U.S. & Canada)

Fax number: **314-447-8029**

**Elsevier Health Sciences Division**
**Subscription Customer Service**
**3251 Riverport Lane**
**Maryland Heights, MO 63043**

*To ensure uninterrupted delivery of your subscription, please notify us at least 4 weeks in advance of move.